Tai Chi Walking for Weight Loss

A Beginner-Friendly Senior Program to Slim Down, Prevent Falls and Regain Independence – Gentle 28-Day Low-Impact Plan, 10 Mins Daily, Zero Equipment

Jing Weston

Disclaimer

This book is intended for general informational and educational purposes only. The exercises and guidance contained in this publication are not a substitute for professional medical advice, diagnosis, or treatment. Always consult your physician or qualified healthcare provider before beginning any new exercise program, particularly if you have a pre-existing medical condition, recent injury, or surgery.

The author and publisher assume no responsibility for any injury, loss, or damage incurred as a result of the use or application of information contained in this book.

Table of Contents

A Note from the Author

There is a specific moment I have watched happen with many of the older adults I have worked with over the years. They are standing at the top of a short flight of steps or at the edge of a curb, and they pause. Not because they cannot manage it. Because they are calculating whether they can. That pause is new. It did not used to be there. And the fact that it is there now changes something about how a person moves through the world.

Walking is the most ordinary thing a person does. It is also, after sixty, one of the things most likely to quietly deteriorate in ways that don't show up until something goes wrong. The stride shortens. The heel strike softens. The moment of single-leg balance in every step, which is what walking actually is, dozens of small balance acts strung together, becomes less confident. Most people don't notice this is happening until they trip on something they would have cleared without thought five years earlier.

I have spent a long time working with older adults on exactly this. On walking. On the quality of the step, the weight transfer, the rhythm of breath through movement. I came to this through Tai Chi, which is built on the same principles: slow deliberate motion, coordinated breath, continuous awareness of where the weight is. What I found, working with people who had fallen, who were afraid of falling, who had given up going to certain places because the ground was uneven or the distance felt uncertain, is that the quality of walking responds to training at any age. Not dramatically. Not overnight. But consistently and reliably.

This program is ten minutes a day. It requires no equipment except a pair of flat, supportive walking shoes. You can do every session indoors if you prefer or need to. The techniques are drawn from Tai Chi footwork and balance training, which means they address the specific mechanics that make walking safer and more efficient: the heel-to-toe weight transfer, the deliberate pace, the hip alignment, the coordination of breath with movement. These are not difficult things. They are precise things. The difference matters.

I want to be honest about what you should expect. You may not be walking longer distances by Day 28 than you are now. What you will likely be doing is walking more deliberately, with more control over each step, and with more confidence in what your body can manage. That improvement in quality is worth more than any increase in distance, because quality is what prevents falls. Quality is also what allows the body to burn fat from walking in a way that distracted, anxious walking does not. The slow deliberate pace, with coordinated breath, is where both benefits live.

The program builds gradually. Week One establishes two foundational techniques and asks nothing more. By Week Four, you will be working through the complete set of six techniques with outdoor terrain options available. The daily sessions are coached, not just described. Each day entry includes a specific note from me about what to focus on. Walking in a quiet space with something precise to pay attention to is a different practice from walking distracted. The focus is part of what makes it work.

One more thing before you start. This program is for people who walk or who want to walk again. It is not for those looking to push their distance or speed. It is for people who have become cautious, who have shortened their outings, who hold on to walls and furniture in ways they didn't used to. Those people are the ones this program was designed around, and those are the changes it is designed to produce.

You don't need to be in good shape to start. You need to be willing to show up for ten minutes and pay attention to how you move. That is all.

Jing Weston

Before You Begin

There are a few things worth settling before we proceed. None of them take long. All of them matter.

Medical Disclaimer

Please speak with your doctor before starting this program. This is especially important if you have experienced a fall in the past year, if you have a diagnosed balance disorder, if you have had lower-body surgery within the past twelve months, if you have peripheral neuropathy, or if you have been advised to limit weight-bearing activity for any reason.

Tai Chi walking is low-impact and designed for older adult beginners. It is among the safest forms of movement available for this population. That said, walking involves periods of single-leg balance with every step, which means there is always some fall risk, particularly early in the program when the techniques are new. The Pre-Walk Body Check in Chapter Three reduces this risk significantly. Do not skip it.

If you experience dizziness, sharp joint pain, significant breathlessness, or any sensation that feels wrong during a session, stop. Rest. Consult your doctor before continuing. Pain that is sharp or joint-specific is different from normal tiredness or mild muscle soreness that comes from using legs and hips in a more deliberate way. Learn to distinguish between the two.

This book does not treat, cure, or diagnose any medical condition. It is a walking program for educational purposes. Your health decisions are your own and should be made in consultation with people who know your medical history.

What You Need

The full list is short.

Walking shoes. Flat, supportive, well-fitting shoes with non-slip soles. Not sandals. Not slippers. Not thick-soled running shoes with heavy cushioning that reduces ground feel. Canvas shoes, light trainers, or purpose-made walking shoes all work well. The sole should be firm enough to support the foot and thin enough to feel the ground underfoot. If you have orthotics, wear them.

A clear floor space. For indoor practice, roughly ten feet of unobstructed walking room. A hallway, a cleared living room, or a bedroom with furniture moved to one side. The floor should be non-slip. Thick carpet makes heel-to-toe walking difficult and should be avoided in the first two weeks. Wood floor, tile, or low-pile carpet is ideal.

A sturdy chair nearby. Not required for most sessions, but useful in Week One for the balance exercises and the Pre-Walk Body Check. A dining or kitchen chair placed where you can reach it quickly provides a safe reference point while you are building walking confidence.

That is everything. No resistance bands, no foam rollers, no fitness tracker. The program is built around attention to movement, not equipment. A clear space, supportive shoes, and ten minutes of willingness to pay attention is the full requirement.

How to Use This Book

Read Chapter Three before Day 1. It contains the Pre-Walk Body Check, the foundational walking breath, and the three starting baselines that the Day 28 Independence Audit will measure against. Skipping this chapter means skipping the information that makes the program measurable and the assessment meaningful.

Chapter Four is the technique library. Every walking technique in the 28-day program is written out in full here with step-by-step instructions and image prompts. When Chapter Five directs you to a specific technique, come here for the complete instructions. Read through each technique at least once before Day 1. You do not need to memorize them. You need to have seen them.

Chapter Five is the daily program. It tells you what to do each day, in what order, and for how long. Each day's entry is coached, not listed. Read the coaching note before the session. It changes the quality of the practice.

Chapters Six through Eight cover nutrition for walkers, independence beyond the program, and how to interpret the Day 28 results honestly. Read them when they become relevant.

One important note on pace. The techniques in this book are taught more slowly than normal walking. This is deliberate and necessary. The slow pace is where the balance training happens. Moving at your usual pace bypasses the work. If ten minutes of slow deliberate practice feels like more effort than a longer ordinary walk, that is because it is asking more of the specific systems this program is designed to strengthen. Stay with the pace.

A final note on the safety reminders that appear in every technique block. They are not included to frighten you. They are included because specific knowledge of where a technique's fall risk lies is more protective than general caution. A person who knows that the transition from two feet to one foot during a Rooted Step is the moment of highest demand is better prepared for that moment than one who is vaguely worried throughout the entire exercise. Read the safety reminders. They are the most practical sentences in the chapter.

Chapter 1

Walking Changed – But You Can Change It Back

Something shifts in how people walk after sixty. It happens gradually enough that most people don't identify it as a change until someone points it out or until something goes wrong. The stride gets a little shorter. The pace gets a little slower. The confidence in the ground underfoot, which was once automatic, now requires at least a small amount of conscious attention.

None of this is irreversible. But it does not reverse on its own, and it does not reverse without specific practice targeted at the right mechanics.

Why Walking Gets Harder After 60

Walking looks simple from the outside. From the inside, it is one of the most mechanically complex things a human body does. Every step involves a moment of complete single-leg balance, a forward fall caught by the next foot, a chain of weight transfers through the ankle, knee, hip, and spine, and a continuous negotiation between the nervous system and the ground. When all of this is working well, it is invisible. When any part of it starts to slip, the invisibility disappears.

After sixty, several things happen simultaneously that affect gait quality. Muscle mass decreases, particularly in the quadriceps, glutes, and calf muscles that control leg stability. The stride shortens because the leg cannot extend and push off with the same confidence it once had. Proprioception, the body's internal sense of position in space, becomes less precise. The sensory signals from the feet and ankles that tell the brain exactly where the foot is and how the ground is angled arrive more slowly and with less resolution. The brain compensates by taking smaller steps, narrowing the base of the walk, and reducing speed.

These are sensible adaptations. They reduce the demand on a system that is working with less precision. But they also create a feedback loop: reduced movement leads to less practice of the balance systems, which leads to further decline in balance capacity, which leads to more caution and further movement restriction. The person who avoids stairs because they feel uncertain on them becomes less capable on stairs over time. Avoidance, in this context, accelerates the very problem it is trying to manage.

The heel strike is one of the most revealing indicators of gait quality. A confident, functional gait lands on the heel first, rolls through the foot from heel to toe, and pushes off from the toes. After sixty, this pattern commonly softens into what is called a flat-footed gait: the foot comes down more flat, bypassing the heel-to-toe transfer. This shortens the step, reduces push-off power, and significantly reduces the proprioceptive information the foot receives from the ground. Flat-footed walking on uncertain terrain is one of the primary mechanical precursors to falls, because the foot cannot read the surface it is landing on as efficiently.

None of this happens because older adults are careless or inactive. It happens because the specific neural and muscular demands of deliberate quality walking are not built into ordinary daily movement. You can walk to and from the kitchen several times a day and still lose heel-to-toe capacity, because kitchen walking does not ask for it. The practice in this book asks for it specifically. That specificity is what produces the change.

There is one more factor worth naming. Shoe design has changed significantly over the past thirty years, and not entirely in the direction of better gait. Thick-soled running shoes, which are now widely worn for everyday use, reduce ground feel substantially. The proprioceptive signals from the foot that help the brain calibrate each step are muffled by the foam. Walking in thick-soled shoes on familiar terrain is fine. Walking in them on uneven terrain with reduced proprioception is one of the reasons falls happen in conditions that should be manageable.

The changes in walking after sixty are also cumulative in their psychological effect. Each small accommodation, each decision to take the easier route or avoid the unfamiliar surface, reduces not just the physical practice of the avoided movement but the confidence that the movement is possible at all. People often underestimate their physical capacity because their recent experience has been one of avoidance rather than practice. One of the effects of this program, reported consistently by participants, is the discovery that the body is more capable than the preceding months of careful avoidance suggested. The capacity was there. It had not been asked for.

The Fear-Tension Cycle

There is a mechanism that many walking programs do not address, and it may be the most important one for the population this book is written for. It is the relationship between fear of falling and actual fall risk.

The research on this is clear: fear of falling is itself a predictor of falling, independent of physical condition. A person who is afraid of falling walks more tensely, with more muscle activation throughout the leg and trunk than the movement requires. That excess tension impairs the fluid weight transfer that makes gait stable. It makes the body rigid in situations that require adaptability. A tense step on an uneven surface is more likely to trip than a relaxed one, because the relaxed step can absorb the irregularity while the tense step resists it.

Fear also narrows attention. A person focused on not falling watches the ground immediately in front of them rather than maintaining the broader visual field that contributes to balance. The vestibular and visual systems, two of the three inputs the brain uses for balance, function less effectively when attention is narrowed to a single focal point. The paradox is that the more anxiously a person monitors each step, the less reliable their overall balance system becomes.

The grip response is another component of this cycle. When people are afraid of falling, they hold on to things: walls, handrails, furniture, companions. This is sensible as a safety measure. But chronic gripping trains the nervous system to treat walking as a high-risk activity requiring external support, and it reduces the practice time of walking without support. Confidence in unsupported walking cannot be built by avoiding unsupported walking. At some point, in a safe and controlled practice setting, the support must be reduced to allow the body to find its own balance.

The way out of the fear-tension cycle is not reassurance. Telling someone not to worry about falling does not make them less worried about falling. The way out is competence. When a person has practiced the mechanics of a reliable step enough times that the mechanics are trustworthy, the attention that was going toward monitoring danger can return to the environment. The gait relaxes. The balance improves. The fear reduces not because anything was said about the fear, but because the body has been given evidence that it can be relied upon.

This is one of the specific things Tai Chi walking builds. The slow deliberate repetition of the heel-to-toe transfer, the single-leg balance check, the coordinated breath, is practice in trusting the step. Most people find that after two or three weeks of this practice, the quality of their confidence in walking has changed in a way that extends beyond the formal sessions. The walk to the car, the walk through a parking lot, the navigation of an unfamiliar floor surface, all feel different because the body has been practicing competence rather than caution.

What Tai Chi Walking Does

Tai Chi walking is not a faster or longer version of ordinary walking. It is a different quality of the same activity. The distinction is worth being clear about.

Ordinary walking, done at a comfortable automatic pace, does not challenge the balance system very much. The speed and stride length are calibrated by the nervous system to sit within the person's comfortable range. This means the walk feels easy and produces relatively little adaptation in the balance and gait systems. Cardiovascular maintenance and general mobility are real benefits, and they should not be dismissed. But ordinary walking at ordinary pace does not rebuild the specific qualities this book addresses: deliberate weight transfer, confident heel strike, reliable single-leg balance, and coordinated breath.

Tai Chi walking is deliberately slow. Slower than is comfortable for most people initially. This slowness is not a concession to physical limitation. It is the mechanism by which the balance training works. At slow speeds, the nervous system cannot use momentum to carry the body through uncertain phases of the step. Every moment of single-leg balance must be genuinely managed. Every weight transfer must be actively controlled. The slow pace makes visible and trainable the exact mechanics that faster, automatic walking conceals.

The breath coordination adds another layer. Inhaling for two steps and exhaling for two steps in a slow sustained pattern activates the parasympathetic nervous system. Cortisol drops. Muscle tension across the shoulders and hip flexors, where most people carry the physical signature of walking anxiety, begins to soften. The combination of deliberate movement and deliberate breath produces a physiological state that ordinary distracted walking does not.

Proprioceptive training is built into every Tai Chi walking technique. The heel-down, toes-raised pause that begins the Rooted Step is a deliberate proprioceptive cue: the foot is registering the surface, checking for firmness and evenness, before committing the body's weight. This is an instinct that modern smooth flooring and cushioned footwear have made largely unnecessary, and which therefore atrophies. Deliberately practicing it restores the neural pathway. Over weeks, it makes outdoor walking on uneven surfaces less threatening, because the foot is once again reading the ground before loading it.

The arm coordination in Cloud Step and related techniques activates the rotational muscles of the trunk in coordination with the legs. Ordinary walking involves trunk rotation, but most people's rotation has reduced with age, producing a flat upper body and reduced counterbalance for the leg movements. Restoring deliberate arm swing and upper body involvement in the walk improves overall gait efficiency and reduces the energy cost of each step. Many participants report that their back feels better after a few weeks of Tai Chi walking practice because the trunk rotation is re-engaging muscles that had been dormant.

The pace of Tai Chi walking also changes the sensory experience of the environment. Walking slowly enough to notice the ground underfoot, the surface variation, the slight incline of a sidewalk, is a different relationship with the physical world than hurrying through it. This heightened environmental awareness is itself a fall prevention mechanism. Falls often happen partly because the person did not register the relevant information about the surface they were crossing. Tai Chi walking trains the habit of registering it.

Sliming Down and Staying Independent

This book has three stated goals and they are served by the same practice through related but distinct mechanisms.

Walking for fat loss works differently for older adults than standard advice suggests. Moderate-intensity sustained walking, done daily at a pace that allows deliberate breathing, is the optimal condition for fat oxidation in this population. The body preferentially uses fat stores for fuel at low-to-moderate intensity. At higher intensity, glucose becomes the primary fuel source because it can be processed faster. A person walking fast enough to be breathless is burning primarily glucose. A person walking at the slow, deliberate Tai Chi pace with controlled breath is burning primarily fat. The pace is not a compromise. It is the mechanism.

The daily insulin sensitivity window matters as much as the fat oxidation during the walk. In the two to three hours following moderate walking, the muscles of the legs and lower body are significantly more receptive to glucose uptake. Glucose that would otherwise drive insulin secretion and fat storage is instead absorbed by the muscles. Daily practice keeps this window open consistently and the cumulative effect over 28 days shifts the metabolic baseline in a meaningful direction.

Cortisol is the third fat loss mechanism. Rhythmic bilateral movement, the left-right alternation of walking, is one of the most reliable cortisol-lowering activities available. Deliberate slow walking with coordinated breath amplifies this effect through the parasympathetic activation described above. The abdominal fat that many older adults cannot shift despite dietary discipline is frequently being driven by chronically elevated cortisol. Addressing the cortisol rather than only the calories is part of why this walking practice produces body composition changes that conventional approaches do not.

The independence goal operates through the gait and balance improvements described in the sections above. But the two goals reinforce each other practically. A person who is less afraid of falling moves more. They go to more places, accept more invitations to go out, walk more routes. More movement means more daily calorie expenditure, more leg muscle maintenance, better circulation. The improvement in walking quality does not just make the ten-minute session more effective. It changes how much the person moves during the rest of the day, and that cumulative change is as significant as the formal practice.

There is an emotional dimension to the independence goal that deserves plain acknowledgment. For many older adults, the narrowing of their walking range has not been a deliberate choice. It has been a series of accommodations: the longer route avoided because the pavement is uneven, the social event skipped because the parking lot is far, the errand deferred because it involves stairs. Each accommodation is individually reasonable. Together they represent a significant contraction of the person's relationship with the world. This program does not promise to reverse all of that. It does promise to make the first steps of reversal possible, and to give the person a specific reliable practice for building on those steps for as long as they choose to continue.

The relationship between sliming down and staying independent also runs in the other direction. A body carrying less excess weight places less load on the joints with every step.

Less joint load means less discomfort, which means more willingness to walk, which means more practice, which means better balance and gait mechanics. The two goals create a reinforcing cycle when the practice is consistent. The walking makes the sliming easier, and the sliming makes the walking easier. This is why the program does not address them as separate goals requiring separate interventions. They share the same mechanism: ten deliberate minutes daily, with the pace and breath that make both outcomes possible.

People who begin this program often ask how long it will take to notice a difference. The honest answer is that most people notice something within the first week, but not what they expect. They expect to feel lighter or fitter. What they usually notice first is that something about the morning walk to the kitchen feels different. Or the walk across a parking lot. Something in the quality of the movement is different, even if nothing about the appearance or the scale has changed yet. That early qualitative change is the program working. It precedes everything else.

Chapter 2

The Science of the Step

Walking looks like the simplest thing. Physiologically, it is not. This chapter explains what is actually happening inside the body during a deliberate walking session and why ten mindful minutes produces effects that ten distracted minutes does not.

How Walking Burns Fat and Why Pace Matters

The standard instruction for walking and weight loss is to walk faster and farther. For older adults, this is often the wrong advice, and not just because of the joint implications.

Fat oxidation, the process by which the body burns stored fat as fuel, is most efficient at moderate to low exercise intensity. At high intensity, the body switches preferentially to glucose because glucose can be processed faster than fat. A person walking hard enough to breathe heavily is primarily burning glucose. A person walking at a pace that allows slow deliberate breathing is primarily burning fat. For this population, the goal is not to push the heart rate up. It is to sustain the right metabolic state for the duration of the session.

Ten minutes of deliberate Tai Chi walking with breath coordination maintained throughout sustains the fat-oxidizing metabolic state for the entire session. The session is short enough that the body does not shift to glucose dependency, and the breath pattern keeps the respiratory rate controlled. This is not a particularly intense workout. That is exactly the point.

Insulin sensitivity is the other metabolic lever that walking influences. After a moderate walking session, the muscles of the legs and lower body become significantly more receptive to glucose uptake for several hours. Glucose that would otherwise accumulate in the bloodstream and stimulate insulin-driven fat storage is instead absorbed by the muscles. Daily walking keeps this window open consistently. It does not require a long session. It requires a regular one.

The cortisol mechanism is equally important. Chronic low-grade cortisol elevation, common in older adults managing pain, isolation, sleep disruption, or ongoing stress, drives abdominal fat accumulation by altering insulin sensitivity and fat storage patterns. Rhythmic bilateral movement, which walking is, is one of the most reliable cortisol-lowering activities available. The left-right alternation engages both hemispheres of the brain simultaneously and has a documented calming effect on the stress response. Deliberate slow walking with coordinated breath amplifies this effect. The fat loss that follows is partly the result of the walk itself and partly the result of the hormonal environment the walk creates in the hours afterward.

There is also the compounding effect of daily practice on resting metabolic rate. Daily walking, even at low intensity, maintains and gradually rebuilds the leg muscle mass that drives baseline calorie burn. For every pound of functional leg muscle maintained through consistent walking practice, the body burns additional calories at rest each day. Over 28 days this adds up. Over several months it becomes the kind of metabolic shift that makes the body feel different regardless of what the scale reports.

Non-exercise activity thermogenesis, the energy the body uses for all movement that is not formal exercise, also rises with improved walking confidence. A person who is less afraid of walking walks more throughout the day. More spontaneous movement, more trips taken under their own power, more routes navigated that would previously have been driven or avoided. This increase in daily movement accumulates into a meaningful additional calorie expenditure that the ten-minute program itself does not directly account for but consistently produces.

Gait, Gravity, and Where Most Falls Happen

Falls do not usually happen in the dramatic situations people imagine. They do not usually happen on ice, on steep stairs, or in obvious hazard zones. They happen in ordinary places: stepping off a curb, crossing a threshold between two floor surfaces, pivoting to answer the phone, reaching for something while weight is unevenly distributed. They happen in transitions, in the moments between one stable state and another.

The reason falls cluster in these moments is mechanical. A transition requires the body to move through a period of single-leg balance or reduced support, and if the systems managing that balance are working with reduced precision, the transition is when the gap between demand and capacity becomes visible. The step off the curb is not difficult. The brief moment of maximum forward lean before the foot lands is when the fall occurs.

Gravity is always pulling the body toward its center of mass. Walking is a controlled process of letting that happen in a forward direction, step by step. The body's center of mass moves slightly forward during each step, and each foot placement catches it. When foot placement is late, imprecise, or lands on an unexpected surface, the center of mass continues forward without being caught. That is what a fall is, mechanically. Not a dramatic event. A timing gap.

Tai Chi walking trains transitions specifically. The Rooted Step slows the heel-strike moment down enough that the foot can assess the surface before weight is loaded. The Pivot Turn addresses the indoor rotation that produces so many falls when done casually. The Side-Open Step trains lateral weight transfer. Each technique addresses a specific class of transition that ordinarily goes unexamined. After weeks of deliberate practice, these transitions become more reliable not because the person is more careful in the moment, but because the body has built the specific neural and muscular patterns that execute them more precisely.

The visual component of fall prevention deserves mention. Many older adults develop a habit of watching their feet while walking. This is intuitive: if you are uncertain about footing, looking at your feet seems like it should help. In practice, watching your feet deprives the visual system of the forward view it needs to anticipate the next obstacle. The instruction to keep the gaze forward at eye height, which appears in every Tai Chi walking technique in this book, is not aesthetic. It is a balance intervention. The eyes need to read ahead because foot placement is managed by the proprioceptive system, not the visual one.

Leg Strength, Hip Stability, and the Independence Connection

The quadriceps muscles at the front of the thigh are the primary muscles responsible for controlling the descent of body weight onto a forward foot. They act as brakes during the weight transfer, preventing the knee from buckling. After sixty, the quadriceps decline faster than almost any other major muscle group. The result is a gait that becomes hesitant at the point of loading: the step becomes smaller, the foot placement flatter, the weight transfer faster and less controlled, because the muscle managing the transfer cannot provide sufficient resistance.

Tai Chi walking rebuilds quadriceps function through the slow, controlled weight transfers of every technique. The Rooted Step performed slowly asks the quadriceps to manage body weight through the full range of the transfer rather than allowing a quick flat-footed drop. Done daily over four weeks, this produces measurable improvement in the muscle's capacity to control the loading phase of each step.

Hip stability is the other major determinant of independent walking. The gluteus medius on the outer hip prevents the pelvis from tilting sideways when one leg is off the ground. When this muscle is weak, the hip drops on the unsupported side with each step, reducing the precision of foot placement. The slow weight shifts in Tai Chi walking, particularly in the Side-Open Step and Cloud Step, directly train the hip stabilizers by requiring the pelvis to stay level during deliberate lateral transfers. A person who practices these techniques for three weeks will feel the hip stabilizers in ways that ordinary walking pace does not produce.

The independence connection is direct. The ability to stand up from a chair, climb stairs, navigate a shopping aisle, carry a bag, and respond to an unexpected surface all depend on leg strength and hip stability more than any other physical factor. A person whose legs can control a slow deliberate step can manage the demands of daily life more reliably than one whose legs are only strong enough for a rapid flat-footed walk. The program builds the specific capacity that transfers.

Ankle strength and mobility complete the picture. The ankle is the first joint to receive impact in every step and the last joint to push off. Ankle mobility determines how far forward the shin can travel over the foot during the weight transfer, which determines the stride length. Ankle strength determines how much power the push-off produces. Both decline with age and limited movement. The deliberate heel-to-toe practice in the Rooted Step and Heel-to-Toe Transfer techniques in Chapter Four specifically address ankle range of motion and the small calf and shin muscles that control ankle movement in both directions.

The interaction between leg strength, hip stability, and ankle control is cumulative and interconnected. A weakness in any one of the three reduces the reliability of the entire chain. A hip that tilts during the single-leg phase of the step puts extra load on the knee. A knee that cannot absorb that load transfers stress to the ankle. An ankle that lacks the strength to manage the stress shortens the step. Tai Chi walking addresses all three simultaneously through the same slow deliberate practice, which is one reason the functional improvements that participants notice tend to appear across multiple areas at once rather than in a single isolated muscle group.

What Your Body Gains From 10 Minutes a Day

Ten minutes seems like a small amount of time. The physiological case for its adequacy is worth making clearly.

The nervous system adaptation that produces improved gait quality does not require long sessions. It requires frequent, precise repetitions of the target pattern. The brain learns movement through repetition, not duration. Ten minutes of precise, slow, deliberate walking practice daily produces more neural adaptation in the specific gait patterns being trained than an hour of automatic walking once a week. Frequency and precision are the variables that matter. Duration and intensity are not the primary factors here.

The metabolic effects described above, fat oxidation, insulin sensitivity, cortisol reduction, all activate within the first few minutes of moderate-intensity movement and continue into the hours that follow. A ten-minute session opens these metabolic windows. A longer session does not produce proportionally larger effects. What a longer session does produce is more fatigue and more recovery demand, both of which can make daily practice harder to sustain. The ten-minute target is not a concession to limited capacity. It is the optimal duration for daily adaptation without compromising the ability to practice again the following morning.

The cumulative effect of daily practice is the argument. One session produces small changes. Seven sessions produce a pattern of neural and metabolic adaptation. Twenty-eight sessions produce changes in muscle capacity, gait quality, and hormonal baseline that are genuinely measurable and that extend well beyond the formal practice time. The people who complete this program consistently report improvements in morning stiffness, ease of walking in public, and confidence on stairs. They are not surprised that the program helped. They are surprised by how much, given the brevity of each session.

The final thing ten mindful minutes provides is something harder to quantify. A person who spends ten minutes each morning paying deliberate attention to how they move carries that attention, in reduced form, through the rest of the day. The heel-to-toe awareness does not switch off when the session ends. It seeps into the walk to the car, the walk through the grocery store, the navigation of the parking lot. That carry-over is why the improvements participants report in daily walking confidence seem disproportionate to the daily session. The practice builds a capacity that operates continuously, not only during the ten minutes.

This is also why consistency matters more than intensity in this program. Missing a session here and there has less effect on the outcome than practicing at too high a pace. The neural adaptation requires repetition. The metabolic adaptation requires regularity. Both are best served by showing up for ten minutes every morning at the pace and attention level the techniques require. That is the full prescription. Nothing else needs to be added to it.

Chapter 3

Walk Before You Walk

The ten minutes before your first session matter more than most people expect. Getting them right does not take long. Skipping them is where most early problems start.

Clearing Space – Indoors, Outdoors, and in Between

The first decision this program asks you to make is where you will walk. The answer matters more in Week One than at any other point, because you are learning new mechanics in a setting you cannot yet fully predict. A space that works well for ordinary walking may not work as well for the slow, deliberate, attention-intensive walking this program uses.

For indoor practice, you need an unobstructed path of at least ten feet. A hallway is ideal. A cleared corridor through the living room or bedroom works equally well. The critical factor is that the path should be genuinely clear, meaning no rugs with curled edges, no extension cords crossing the floor, no objects at ankle height that are not immediately obvious. At the pace Tai Chi walking uses, your attention will be on your body mechanics rather than on floor hazards, and the environment needs to support that shift of attention.

Floor surface matters in the first two weeks. Thick pile carpet requires more ankle work and masks the heel-to-toe feedback the techniques are designed to produce. Smooth tile or hardwood is ideal. Low-pile carpet is acceptable. If your available indoor space is thickly carpeted throughout, work in the space that has the lowest pile. The techniques will still function, but progress the floor difficulty gradually rather than beginning on the most challenging surface.

For outdoor practice, which becomes available from Week Three onward, a flat paved surface with predictable footing is the starting point. A sidewalk in a quiet residential area, a paved path in a park, a flat car park at an off-peak hour. The surface should be familiar enough that you are not navigating its unpredictability and learning the techniques simultaneously. Save uneven terrain for when the techniques themselves are secure, which happens around Day 18 to 21 for most people.

A sturdy chair positioned at the edge of your practice space is useful in Weeks One and Two, not for leaning on continuously, but as a reference point. Knowing it is there reduces the background tension that some people carry when practicing balance-demanding movement in an open space. As confidence builds, the chair's presence becomes less relevant. By Week Three most people have stopped thinking about where it is.

Footwear, Grip, and Surface Awareness

The shoe instruction from the "Before You Begin" section is revisited here in more specific terms.

The ideal shoe for this program has a flat or very slightly raised heel, a firm but not rigid sole, and enough interior support to prevent the foot from rolling inward or outward under the body's weight. It fits snugly enough that the foot does not slide inside the shoe during the weight transfer. The sole material should provide traction on the floor surface you are using without gripping so firmly that pivoting becomes difficult.

What you are avoiding: thick cushioned running shoes, because they reduce ground feel and proprioceptive feedback. Sandals and backless shoes, because the foot cannot be controlled accurately within them. Socks on smooth surfaces without grip, because the combination produces exactly the sliding conditions that generate falls. Shoes with worn or uneven soles, because the foot will compensate for the worn area in ways that interfere with the heel-to-toe mechanics you are trying to train.

Grip awareness is the habit of noticing how the surface you are walking on relates to the grip your shoes provide. Before each outdoor session, a two-second assessment of the surface: is it wet, is it sandy or gritty, is there a transition between surface types coming up? This is not anxious monitoring. It is the same environmental reading that experienced walkers do automatically. You are making it deliberate until it becomes automatic.

Indoor grip awareness focuses on transitions: carpet to tile, mat to hardwood, room to room. These are where traction changes unexpectedly. Note them before the session and plan to slow down slightly at each one.

The Pre-Walk Body Check

This three-minute routine is performed before every session, not just in Week One. It identifies areas of discomfort that need accommodation and brings attention into the body before the walk begins. The transition from ordinary morning awareness to the quality of attention the techniques require starts here.

Ankle Mobility Check:

1. Stand in your clear floor space with feet hip-width apart. Lightly rest one hand on a wall or chair back if needed.

2. Lift your right heel slowly from the floor, rising onto the ball of the right foot. Move through the full comfortable range without forcing it.

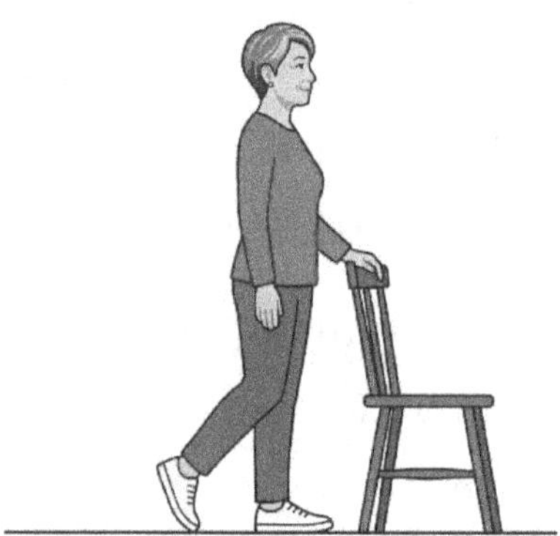

3. Lower the heel with control. Note whether the ankle feels stiff, limited, or comfortable. Do not push through sharp discomfort.

4. Repeat on the left side. Complete three gentle rises on each side.

Knee Comfort Check:

1. Stand with both feet flat and hip-width apart. Bend both knees gently to a shallow squat, roughly fifteen degrees, as if beginning to sit down.

2. Hold for two counts. Note any sharpness, clicking, or significant restriction.

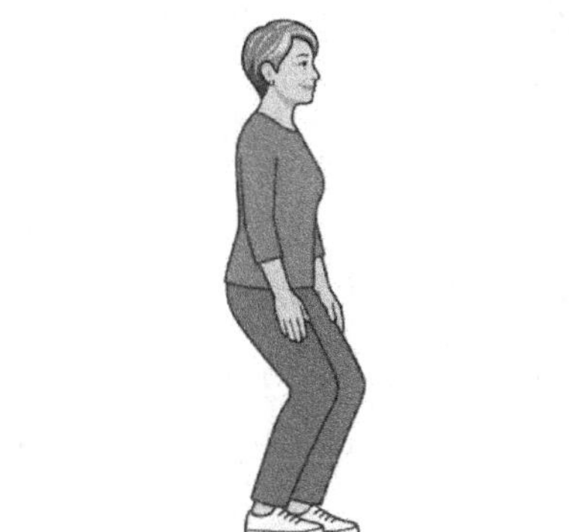

3. Return to standing slowly. If the knee check reveals sharp pain, reduce the range or skip the knee-bending in today's session and work with a shallower weight transfer.

Hip Flexibility Check:

1. Stand with one hand on the chair back. Lift your right knee gently to hip height, or as high as is comfortable, and hold for two counts.

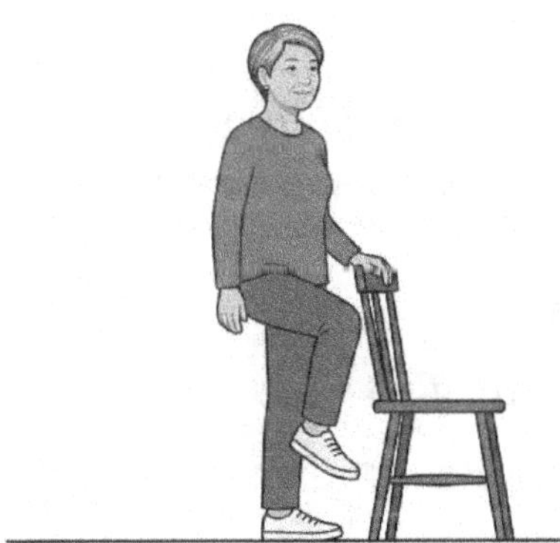

2. Lower the right foot. Lift the left knee in the same way. Note any restriction, tightness, or asymmetry between sides.

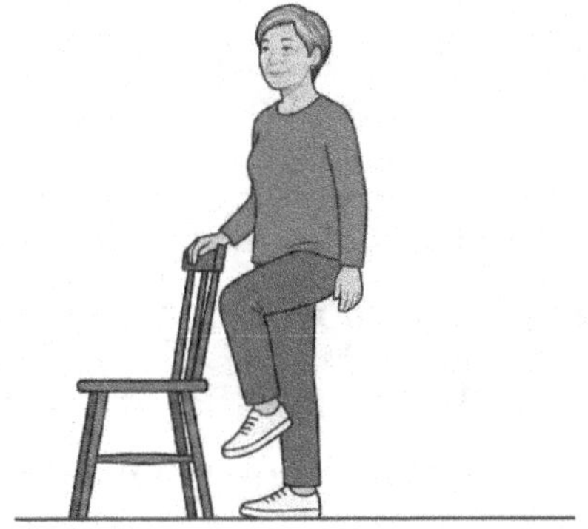

3. Complete two lifts on each side. The hip check reveals which side may need more accommodation in the lateral weight transfer techniques today.

Balance Check:

1. Stand with feet together and arms at your sides. Release the chair.

2. Hold the standing position for ten seconds. Notice whether the weight feels evenly distributed or whether there is a tendency to drift to one side.

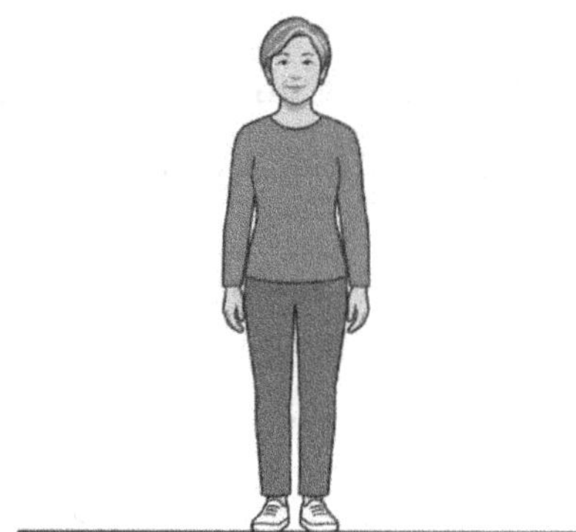

3. If balance today feels less stable than usual, keep the chair within arm's reach throughout the session and use the chair-assisted modifications for any technique that challenges balance.

Bad Knees, Hip Pain, and Uneven Ground

Pain is information. The distinction that matters is between the kind of discomfort that signals productive work and the kind that signals something requiring accommodation.

General morning stiffness in the knees or hips that eases within the first few minutes of movement is normal for this population and is not a reason to stop or reduce the session. The Pre-Walk Body Check and the early steps of the session produce the movement that resolves it. Stay with the program.

Sharp, stabbing, or joint-specific pain that appears during a particular movement is a different signal. Reduce the range of that movement to find a version that is uncomfortable in the productive sense rather than in the stop signal sense. Every technique in Chapter Four has guidance for reducing the demand of the movement while preserving the core mechanic. Use it.

Hip pain during the lateral weight transfers of the Wave Step or Side-Open Step usually indicates that the transfer is moving faster than the hip stabilizers can manage. Slowing down further and reducing the lateral range until the hip is comfortable is the adjustment. The hip stabilizer work is the point of those techniques. If the hip cannot manage the full range, it simply means the technique is asking exactly the right question and needs more practice time before the range increases.

Uneven ground outdoors should be introduced in Week Three after the fundamental techniques are secure. When you do introduce it, reduce the overall pace further and shorten the session duration slightly. Walking on uneven ground with good technique is more demanding than walking on a flat surface. It is also more directly applicable to real-world independence. Build toward it deliberately rather than avoiding it indefinitely.

Your Baseline Walk Test

Before Day 1, take three measures and write them down. They are the starting point against which the Day 28 Independence Audit is measured.

Measure one: comfortable walking distance. Walk at your ordinary comfortable pace on a flat surface indoors or outdoors. Walk until you choose to stop. Note the approximate distance and how the walk felt. You are establishing what comfortable ordinary walking looks like for you today, not trying to walk as far as possible.

Measure two: single-leg balance hold. Stand near a wall or chair. Lift one foot slightly off the floor and count how long you can hold before needing to touch down or grab support. Try both sides. Write down the approximate times. You are establishing a baseline, not a score.

Measure three: stiffness level on waking. For three mornings before Day 1, rate your leg and lower body stiffness on waking on a scale of one to five. One is no stiffness, five is significant stiffness that limits movement until it eases. Average the three readings.

Keep these three numbers somewhere accessible. The Day 28 Independence Audit at the end of Chapter Five will return to each of them with specific questions. They are the most honest measure of what this program has done for your body.

The Foundational Breath

Walking breath coordination from Tai Chi is simple in description and requires practice to integrate. It is worth establishing it here, before Day 1, because it underpins every technique in the program. The breath pattern is: inhale for two steps, exhale for two steps.

Each inhale is through the nose, slow and deliberate, expanding the belly outward before the chest rises. Each exhale is through slightly parted lips, longer than the inhale, allowing the belly to draw gently inward. This is diaphragmatic breathing, the same pattern described in Chapter Three of the foundational Tai Chi books, here applied to walking.

Foundational Walking Breath

The breath that coordinates with every walking technique in this program. Establishing it before Day 1 means it is available automatically from the first session.

Starting Position:

Stand in your practice space. Feet hip-width apart, weight centered, knees soft. Both arms hanging at your sides.

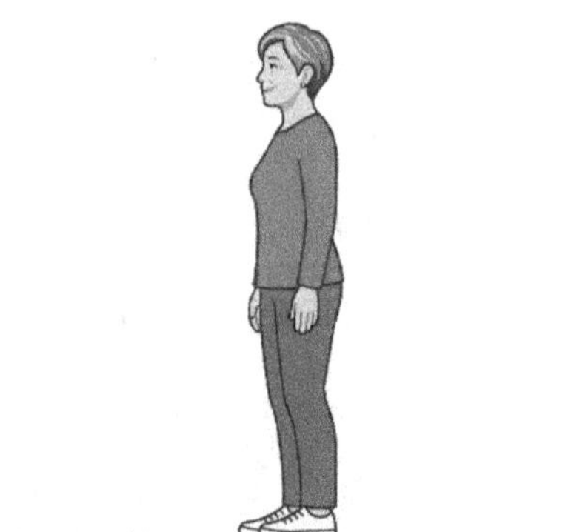

Steps:

1. Begin walking forward at a very slow pace. Each step is deliberate, heel landing first.
2. As the right heel lands, begin a slow inhale through the nose. Count the step: one.

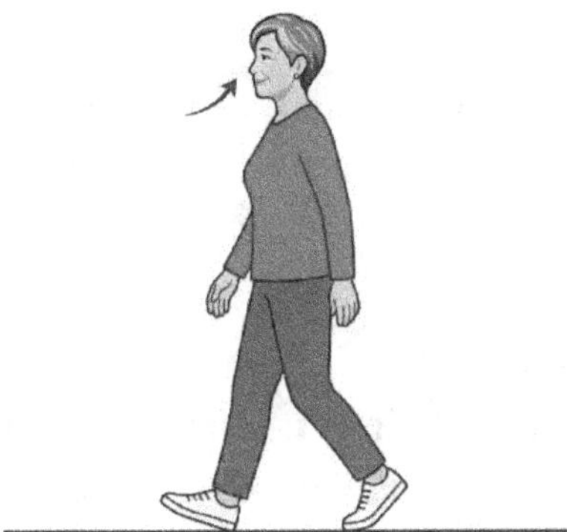

3. As the left heel lands, continue the inhale. Count: two.

4. As the right heel lands again, begin a slow exhale through slightly parted lips. Count: three.

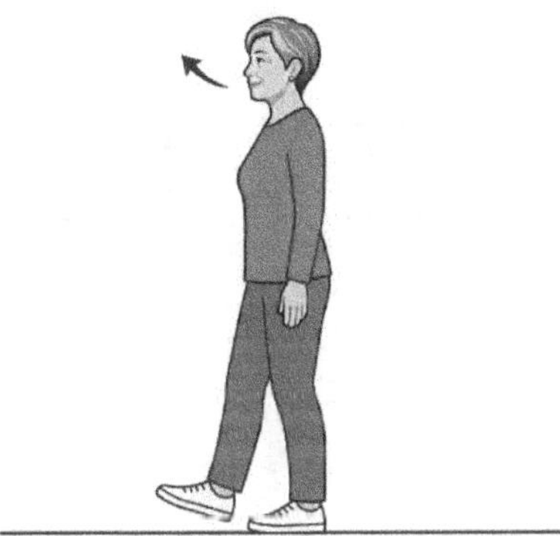

5. As the left heel lands, continue the exhale and allow it to complete gently. Count: four.

6. Continue for eight to ten steps at this pace, maintaining the two-step inhale, two-step exhale pattern.

7. If the breath pattern and the steps do not synchronize immediately, slow down further rather than rushing the breath to catch the steps.

BREATHING: The breath drives the pace, not the other way around. If you find yourself hurrying the steps to keep up with the breath, slow the steps down.

FEEL IT: After four or five complete breath cycles, a quieting sensation across the chest and shoulders. The walk begins to feel different from ordinary walking. That shift is the parasympathetic activation the program depends on.

CHAIR-ASSISTED MODIFICATION
Practice the foundational breath seated. Sit at the front of your chair, spine upright. March the feet gently in place, lifting each heel alternately. Inhale for two marches, exhale for two marches. The coordination is identical. Build it seated, then transfer it to walking.

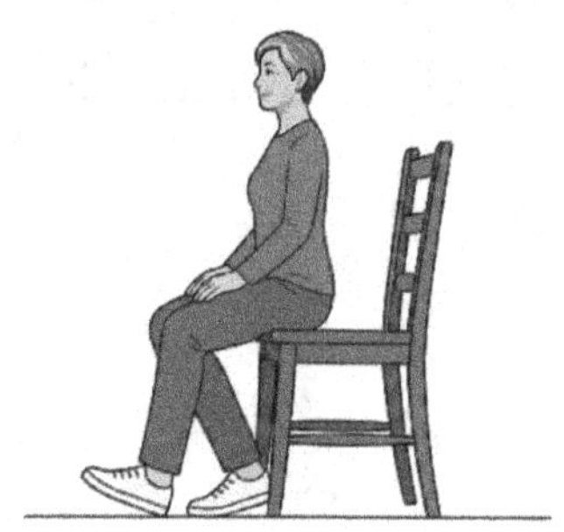

Chapter 4

The Walking Techniques

This is the technique library. Every walking form in the 28-day program refers back to this chapter for complete instructions. Read through all six techniques before Day 1. You do not need to memorize them. You need a map of the territory.

The Balance Builders at the end of this chapter appear in the program from Week Three onward. They are separate from the walking techniques but built on the same principles.

Reading the Technique Blocks

Every technique in this chapter follows the same layout. The starting position is described in plain prose, followed by an image showing exactly that position. The numbered steps begin below. Images appear within the step sequence immediately after the step they correspond to, so you can read a step, look at the image, and understand the mechanics before continuing. Each technique ends with three cues and a chair-assisted modification.

The BREATHING cue tells you when to inhale and exhale through the movement. The FEEL IT cue describes what correct practice should feel like in the body. The SAFETY note is the most important sentence in the block. It identifies the specific error or fall risk most associated with that technique. Read it before you practice, not after something goes wrong.

The CHAIR-ASSISTED MODIFICATION is a complete version of the technique with a chair for balance support. It is not a lesser version of the technique. For people whose balance is not yet reliable enough for unsupported walking practice, the chair-assisted modification is the correct version. Practice it until the unsupported version is accessible.

Walking images in this chapter are shown from the side or at a three-quarter angle. Never from the front as the primary view, because foot placement and weight transfer cannot be seen clearly from the front. A ground line appears beneath the feet in every image. This line shows whether the foot is flat, heel-raised, or mid-transfer, which is the most important technical information in a walking technique illustration.

The Core Tai Chi Walking Techniques

Technique 1: The Rooted Step

The foundational movement of the entire program. Trains the heel-to-toe weight transfer that makes every step more deliberate and more stable. This is the technique most people need most and practice least.

Starting Position:

Stand at the beginning of your clear walking path. Feet together, weight centered, knees softly bent. Arms at your sides, shoulders relaxed.

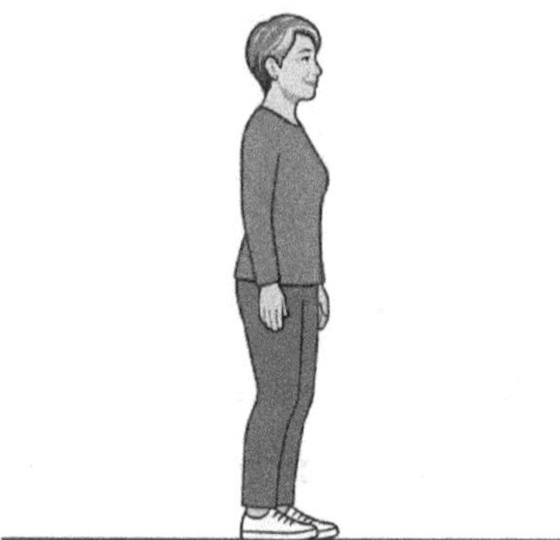

Steps:

1. Shift your weight gently onto the right foot without leaning to the right. The hips stay level.

2. Lift the left foot just barely off the floor and extend it forward, placing the heel down on the ground line first. The toes point upward. The foot has not loaded any weight yet.

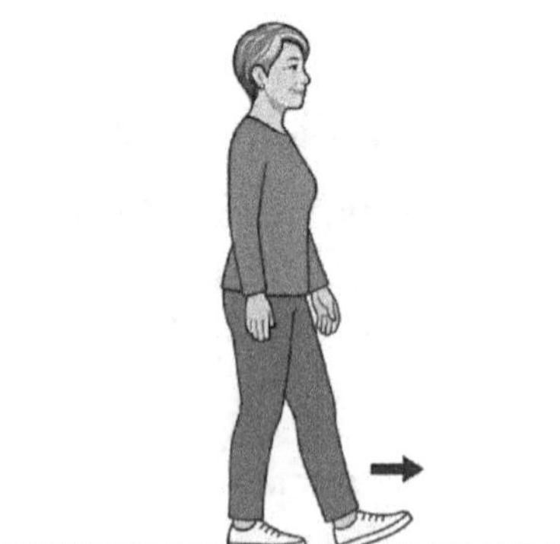

3. Pause for one count with the heel down and toes raised. This is the moment of ground assessment. Feel the surface under the heel.

4. Roll through the foot slowly: heel settles, arch follows, ball contacts, toes come down and then push off gently. Transfer your weight forward as the foot rolls through.

5. As the left foot becomes fully flat, the right heel rises naturally. Do not force it. Let the weight transfer pull the heel up.

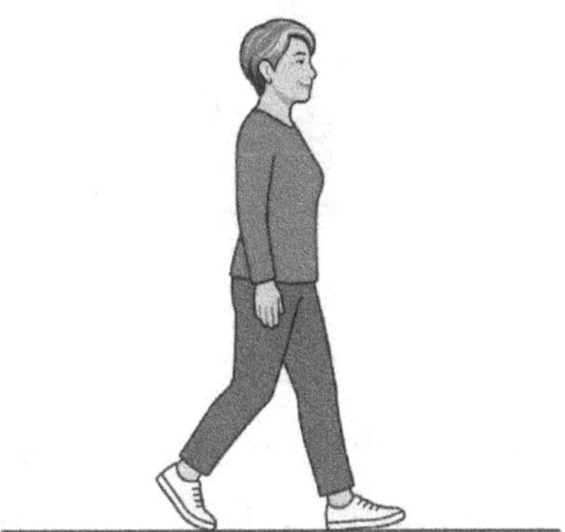

6. Begin the next step: right foot extends forward, heel first, toes up.

7. Continue for the length of your walking path. At the end, turn carefully and return.

BREATHING: Inhale as the heel lands. Exhale as the weight rolls through the foot. This produces one breath per step initially. As the pace settles, the pattern shifts naturally to two steps per inhale and two per exhale.

FEEL IT: A distinct heel contact followed by a rolling sensation through the sole of the foot. The toe push-off at the end of the transfer should feel like a deliberate departure rather than a passive lift.

SAFETY:
The most common error: allowing the heel landing and the weight transfer to happen simultaneously rather than sequentially. The pause after the heel lands is essential. It is where the proprioceptive reading happens. Removing it turns the Rooted Step back into ordinary walking.

CHAIR-ASSISTED MODIFICATION
Hold the back of a chair with both hands. Practice the heel-to-toe roll in place without stepping forward. Lift the right heel while keeping the toes down, then lower it slowly. Alternate feet. This rehearses the transfer mechanics without requiring forward motion or balance management.

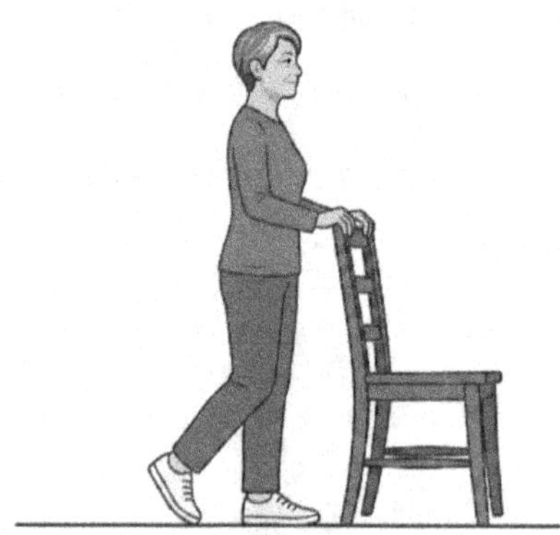

Technique 2: The Tai Chi Pace

Establishes the tempo of the entire program. Not speed. A quality of movement: deliberate, continuous, slightly slower than feels natural. This is where the cortisol regulation and fat oxidation mechanisms operate.

Starting Position:

Begin at the start of your walking path. Use the Rooted Step heel-to-toe mechanics from Technique 1. What changes here is the rhythm and the internal focus.

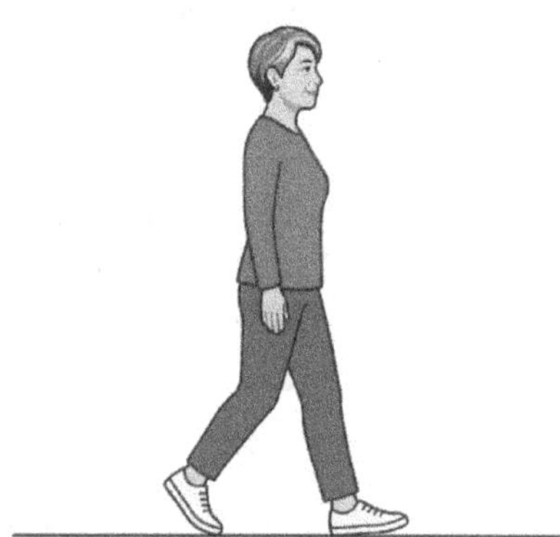

Steps:

1. Begin walking forward using the Rooted Step mechanics. Heel lands first, weight transfers, heel rises at the back.

2. Find the pace where each step takes approximately twice as long as your ordinary walking step. This is the Tai Chi Pace. It will feel uncomfortably slow at first.

3. Allow the arms to swing gently in opposition to the legs: right arm forward as the left leg steps forward. The swing is small and relaxed, not exaggerated.

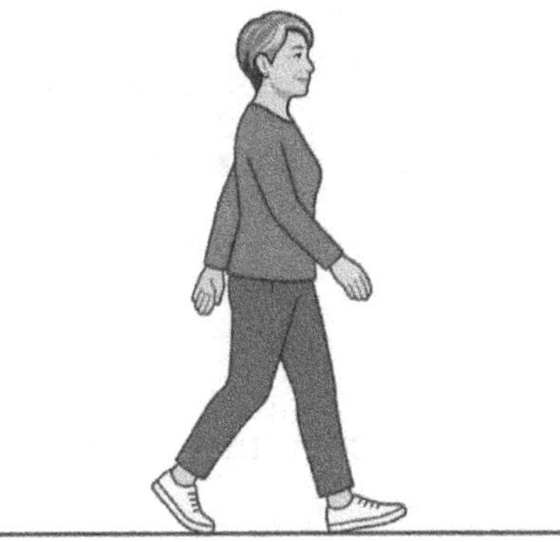

4. Keep the gaze at eye level. Do not look at your feet. The eyes look forward to where you are going.

5. Maintain the two-step inhale, two-step exhale breath pattern from the foundational breath practice.

6. Continue for the duration of the session at this pace. Resist the tendency to speed up when the mechanics feel settled. The pace is the practice.

BREATHING: Two steps inhale, two steps exhale. If the pace slows further, three steps inhale, three exhale. The breath drives the pace.

FEEL IT: A sense of the walk becoming slightly effortful not in the legs but in the attention. Maintaining this pace requires continuous small decisions to stay slow. That quality of sustained attention is the practice.

SAFETY:

The common error is gradual speed increase as the technique becomes familiar. The mechanics feel secure and the pace drifts upward toward ordinary walking speed. Check your pace at the midpoint of each session. If it has increased, reduce it.

CHAIR-ASSISTED MODIFICATION

Practice the Tai Chi Pace tempo while standing in place. March in slow motion, lifting each foot barely off the floor, at the Tai Chi Pace tempo. This rehearses the pace without requiring forward motion and is useful on days when the full walk session is not possible.

Technique 3: Cloud Hands Walking

Adds arm coordination to the walking mechanics. The arms trace slow horizontal arcs while the legs continue the Rooted Step. This technique activates the trunk rotation that improves gait efficiency and counterbalance.

Starting Position:

Begin walking at the Tai Chi Pace. Once the leg mechanics feel settled, begin adding the arm coordination.

Steps:

1. As the left foot steps forward, raise the right arm in a slow arc from the hip to chest height, palm facing left. The left arm descends toward the left hip, palm down.

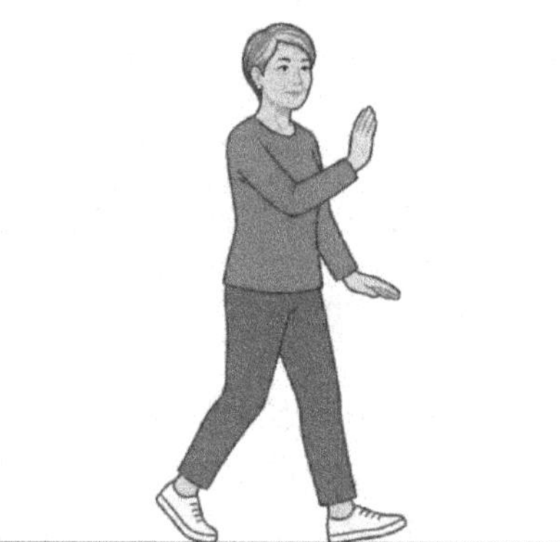

2. As the right foot steps forward, sweep the right arm across the front of the body from right to left, continuing the arc. The gaze follows the right hand.

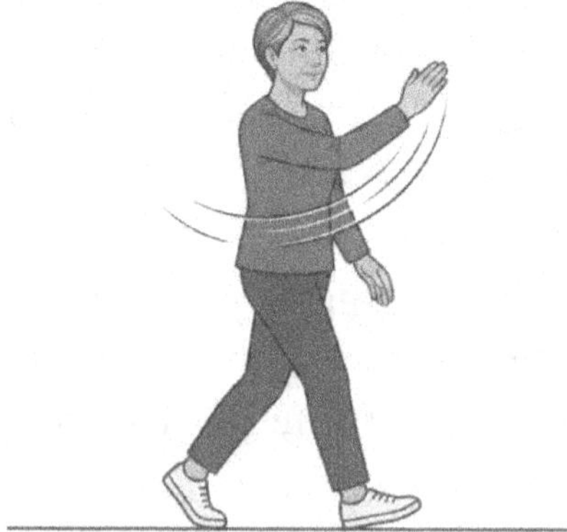

3. As the right arm completes its arc and descends, the left arm rises to chest height and begins its own sweep from left to right.

4. The arms alternate: one rises and sweeps while the other descends. The movement is continuous, no stopping between arcs.

5. Keep the pace of the arms matched to the pace of the steps. Neither rushes the other.

BREATHING: Inhale as each arm rises. Exhale as it sweeps and descends. One full breath per arm cycle.

FEEL IT: A warmth developing across the upper back and through the sides of the waist as the trunk rotation engages. If the arms are moving without any sense of the trunk following them, the rotation has not yet engaged. Slow down further.

SAFETY:
Do not allow the arm movement to pull the upper body off balance. If the arm sweep is causing the torso to lean or the foot placement to become imprecise, reduce the arm arc until the legs and arms can coordinate without either compensating for the other.

CHAIR-ASSISTED MODIFICATION
Practice Cloud Hands Walking from a standing position beside the chair. Hold the chair with one hand for balance. Perform the arm arc with the free arm while stepping gently in place. When the coordination is established, release the chair and perform the full technique.

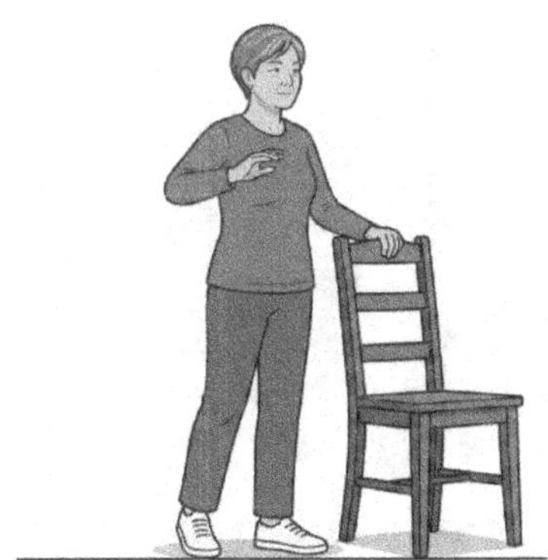

Technique 4: Wave Step

A lateral weight shift exercise that trains the hip stabilizers and the sideways balance mechanics used when navigating confined spaces, crowded aisles, and narrow passages.

Starting Position:

Stand with feet slightly wider than hip-width. Weight centered. Arms at your sides. You will step sideways rather than forward in this technique.

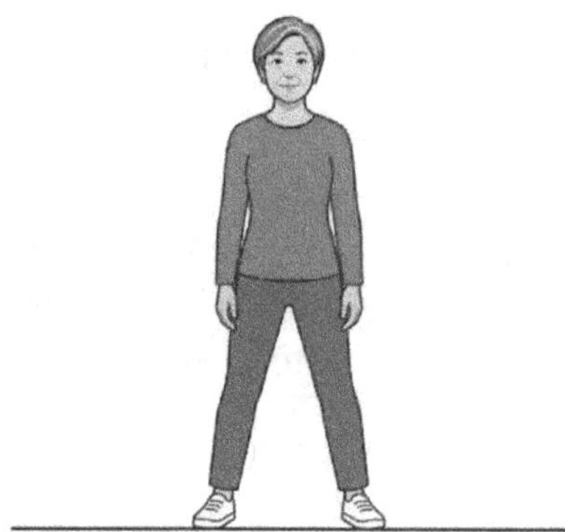

Steps:

1. Shift your weight onto the right foot. Keep the hips level as the weight transfers.

2. Lift the left foot and step it one step further to the left, placing the heel down and then rolling to the full flat foot.

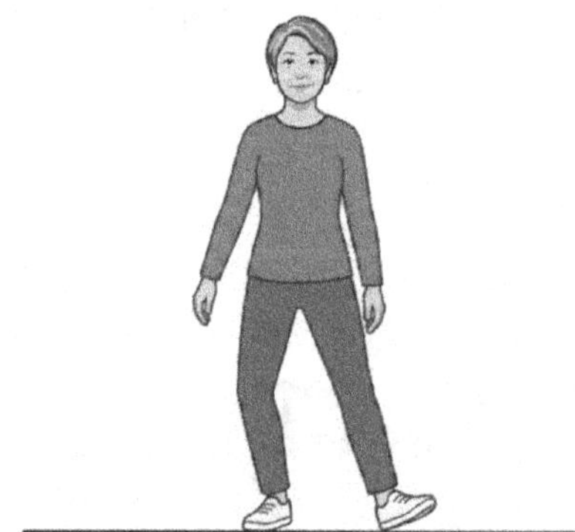

3. Shift your weight onto the left foot as it settles flat. Pause for one count with weight fully on the left.

4. Lift the right foot and bring it to meet the left foot, setting it down flat. Return to the starting position.

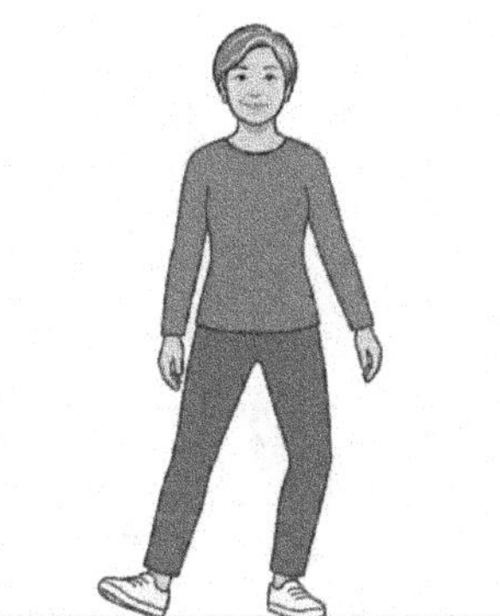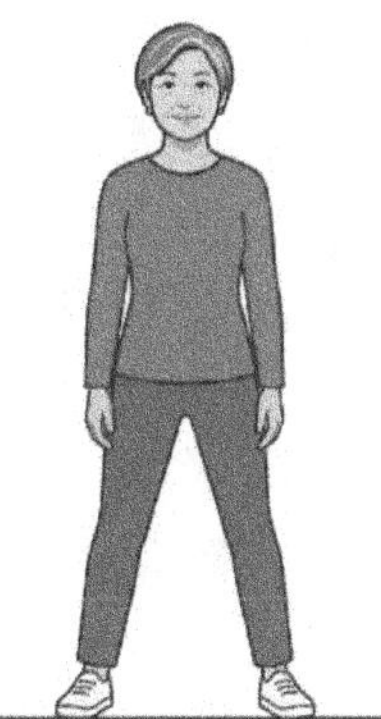

5. Pause for one count. Begin the sequence again: shift right, step left, shift left, close right.

6. Complete eight full cycles moving to the left, then reverse the direction for eight cycles moving to the right.

BREATHING: Inhale as you step out. Exhale as you close.

FEEL IT: A definite engagement in the outer hip of the standing leg as it manages the single-leg phase of the step. This is the gluteus medius working. It should feel like effort, not pain.

SAFETY:
The hips dropping sideways during the step, rather than remaining level, is the primary technique error. It usually means the step is too wide for the current hip stabilizer capacity. Reduce the step width until the hips can maintain level position throughout.

CHAIR-ASSISTED MODIFICATION
Stand behind the chair with both hands on the chair back. Perform the lateral weight shifts and steps with the chair providing forward support throughout. The lateral mechanics are identical. The chair removes the balance demand.

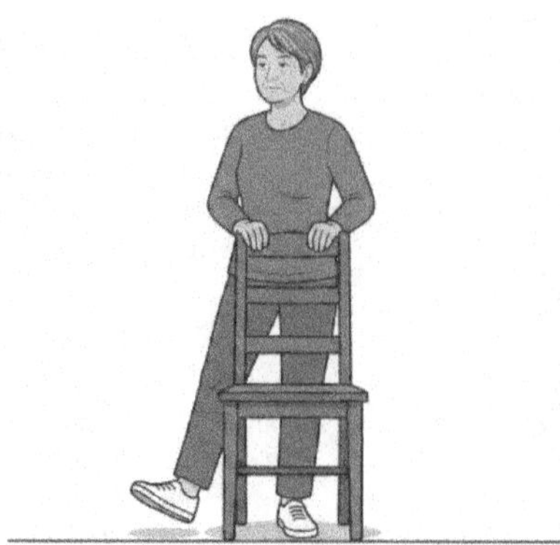

Technique 5: Gathering Walk

A breath-step synchronization technique that deepens the foundational breath pattern established in Chapter Three. The movement slows the walking pace to a meditative tempo while increasing the deliberateness of each weight transfer.

Starting Position:

Begin at the Tai Chi Pace. The Gathering Walk uses the same footwork but adds an arm gathering movement coordinated with the breath.

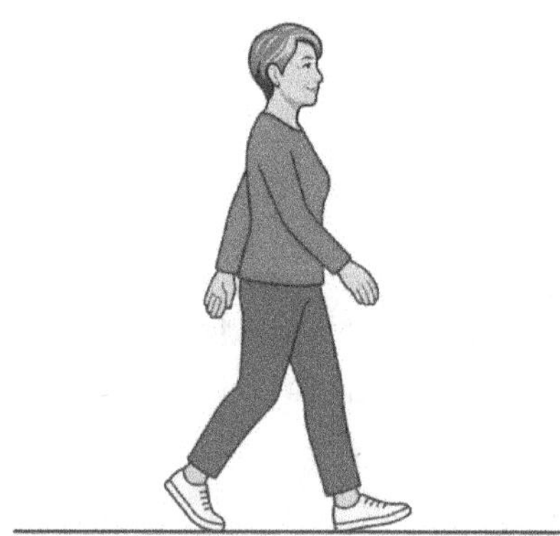

Steps:

1. Take two steps at the Tai Chi Pace. As the second step lands, begin raising both arms slowly from the hips to waist height, palms facing upward. This corresponds to the inhale.

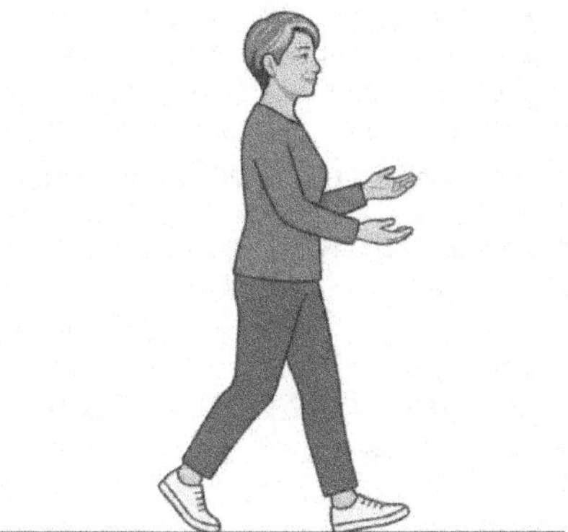

2. Take two more steps. As the third step lands, let the arms continue rising to chest height at their slowest pace.

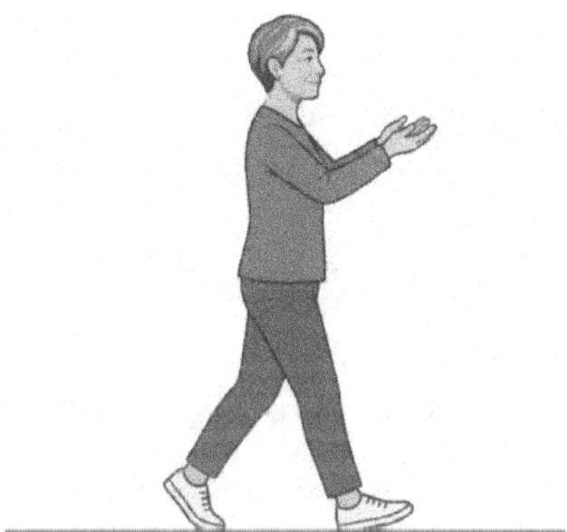

3. As the fourth step lands, begin lowering both arms slowly back toward the hips, palms pressing gently downward. This corresponds to the exhale.

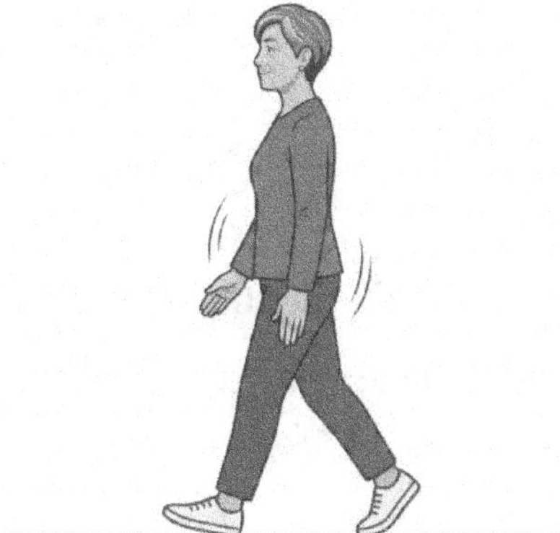

4. Continue the cycle: two steps rising arms, two steps lowering arms, in a continuous slow arc.

5. Maintain the gaze forward throughout. Allow the arm movement to feel like gathering the air in front of you on the inhale and releasing it on the exhale.

6. Continue for the length of your walking path. The Gathering Walk may be used as a transition between more active techniques to restore the breath and slow the pace.

BREATHING: Inhale for the two steps while arms rise. Exhale for the two steps while arms lower. The arms make the breath visible.

FEEL IT: A deepening of the breath with each cycle, as if the arm movement is pulling the breath in more fully than the breath alone would. After three or four cycles, a noticeable reduction in physical tension across the chest and upper back.

SAFETY:
Keep the arm movement light. If the arm raising causes the upper body to lean backward or the weight to shift behind the center of gravity, reduce the height of the arm raise. The arms should feel almost weightless throughout.

CHAIR-ASSISTED MODIFICATION
Practice the Gathering Walk arm movement while seated. Sit at the front of your chair and step the feet gently in place at the Tai Chi Pace tempo. Raise and lower the arms in the same coordinated pattern. The breath integration is identical seated or standing.

Technique 6: Closing Walk

The deceleration technique that ends every practice session. It signals to the nervous system and the body that the active portion is complete. Every session ends with the Closing Walk. Without exception.

Starting Position:

You are continuing the session's final walk at whatever pace it has reached. The Closing Walk begins with a deliberate reduction of pace over the final two minutes of the session.

Steps:

1. Allow the pace to reduce over four to six steps until you reach the slowest comfortable walking speed, slower than the Tai Chi Pace if possible.

2. Continue at this pace for eight to ten steps, allowing the breath to slow with the movement.

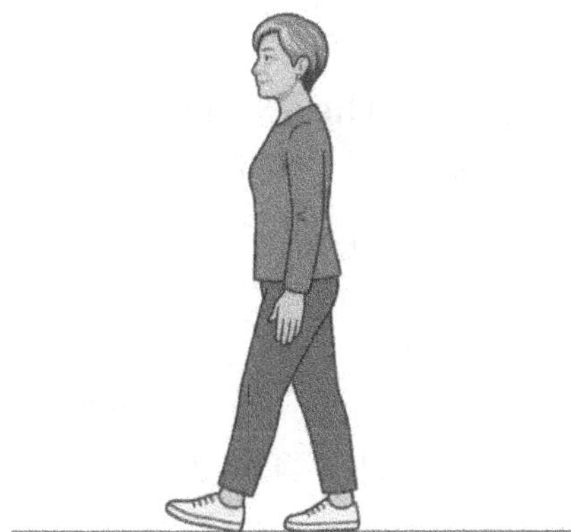

3. At the end of the walking path, come to a natural stop. Stand with feet hip-width apart and weight centered.

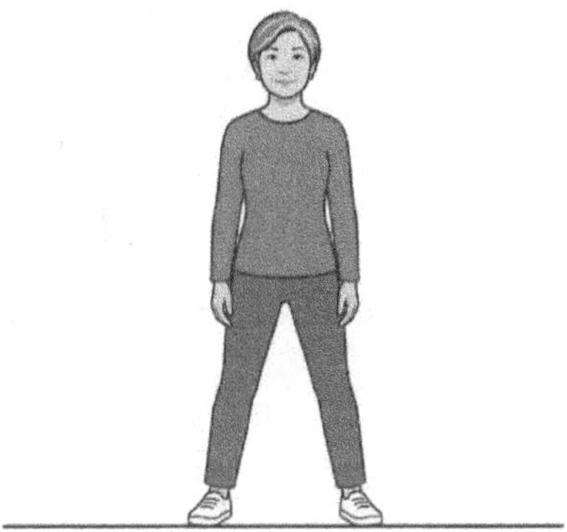

4. Complete three full breathing cycles: inhale for four counts, exhale for six counts. Do not rush.

5. Notice the quality of the body after the session. Compared to how it felt before the Pre-Walk Body Check, what has changed?

BREATHING: The exhale is longer than the inhale throughout. Four counts in, six counts out. The extended exhale is what completes the parasympathetic activation.

FEEL IT: A settling sensation through the legs and lower body. Some people feel warmth in the feet and calves. The breath should feel slower and more spacious than it did at the start of the session.

SAFETY:
Do not stop abruptly from a walking pace. The deceleration is part of the technique. An abrupt stop after sustained walking can cause a brief blood pressure drop in some older adults. The gradual slowdown prevents this.

CHAIR-ASSISTED MODIFICATION
If the session was conducted primarily with the chair, finish by sitting at the front of the chair and completing the three breathing cycles. The closing intention is the same whether standing or seated.

Arm Coordination and Upper Body Alignment

Before the Balance Builders, a brief note on the arm and upper body principles that run through all six techniques. The arms in Tai Chi walking are not passengers. They are counterweights. As the right leg steps forward, the left arm swings gently forward. This opposition reduces the rotational load on the spine and makes the gait more efficient. As the pace slows, the arm swing also slows. At the Tai Chi Pace, the swing is barely perceptible from the outside but clearly felt from within.

The head position is equally important and frequently neglected. The head should sit level over the shoulders, chin neither raised nor dropped, gaze at eye level ahead. A dropped chin compresses the cervical spine and reduces the visual field needed for environmental awareness. A raised chin shifts the center of gravity backward and reduces the security of the heel strike. Level chin, gaze forward: this is the constant through every technique.

Turning, Stopping, and Navigating Obstacles Safely

Turns are where many falls happen, because the rotational demand on the hip and ankle exceeds the linear walking demand. The Tai Chi walking turn uses a pivot rather than a swing: the weight transfers fully onto one foot, and the free foot steps to the new direction in a small deliberate step rather than a sweeping arc. For indoor practice at the end of a walking path, pivot on the ball of the leading foot rather than spinning on the heel.

Stopping safely means decelerating before coming to rest, as the Closing Walk technique establishes. The instinct to stop suddenly when something unexpected appears, a sound, a door opening, needs to be replaced by a trained deceleration. Practice stopping intentionally at various points in the session, not just at the end, to build the habit.

Obstacles in real-world walking, a curb, a step, a piece of furniture, require a modified Rooted Step with a higher foot clearance and a more deliberate pause at the top of the obstacle before weight transfer. This is practiced in Week Three when outdoor walking is introduced. Until then, the indoor environment should be arranged to remove the need to navigate around obstacles.

Balance Builders

These four exercises appear in the 28-day program beginning in Week Three. They are performed at the end of the walking session, before the Closing Walk. Each one addresses a specific balance mechanism that transfers directly to safer walking.

Balance Builder 1: Standing Heel Raise

Strengthens the calf muscles and small ankle stabilizers that control the push-off phase of every step and that are the primary deficit in flat-footed walking.

Starting Position:

Stand behind your chair with both hands resting lightly on the chair back. Feet hip-width apart, flat on the floor.

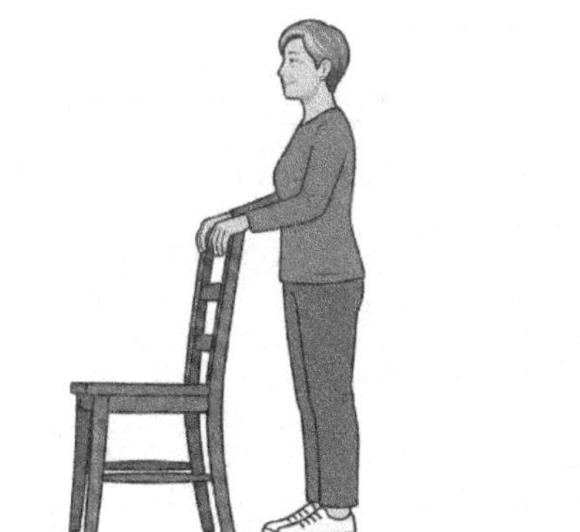

Steps:

1. Rise slowly onto the balls of both feet, lifting the heels off the floor. Keep the weight even across both feet.

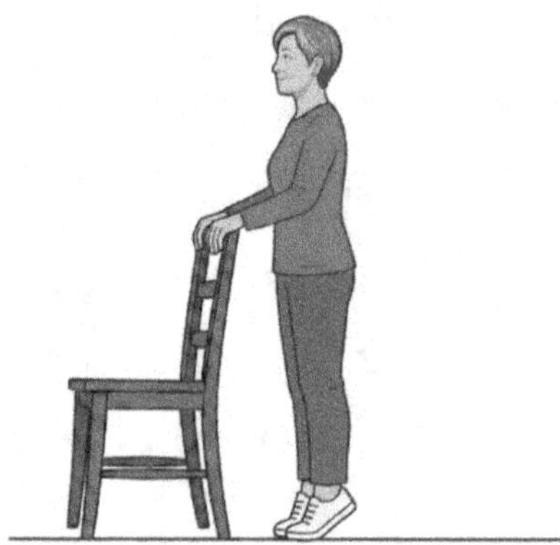

2. Hold at the top for two counts. Do not grip the chair.

3. Lower the heels slowly and with complete control back to the floor.

4. Complete 10 repetitions at a slow deliberate pace.

BREATHING: Inhale as you rise. Exhale as you lower.

FEEL IT: A clear engagement in the calf muscles from repetition five or six onward. This is the work that builds the push-off power.

> **SAFETY:**
> Do not allow the ankles to roll outward at the top of the rise. Keep the weight centered across the ball of each foot.

Balance Builder 2: Single-Leg Stand

Directly trains the single-leg balance phase that occurs with every walking step. The most specific balance exercise available for gait improvement.

Starting Position:

Stand beside your chair with one hand available to touch it. Feet hip-width apart.

Steps:

1. Shift your weight fully onto the left foot without leaning to the left.

2. Lift the right foot just a few inches off the floor. Do not touch the chair unless needed.

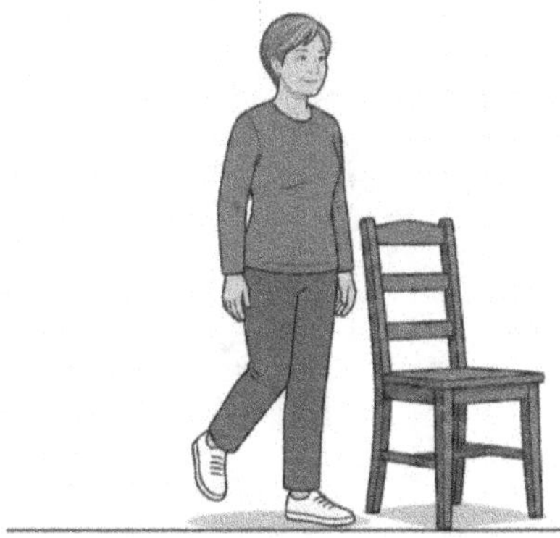

3. Hold for up to 15 seconds, building toward 30 seconds over the program.

4. Lower the right foot and repeat on the other side.

5. Complete three holds on each side.

BREATHING: Breathe naturally. Do not hold the breath during the balance hold.

FEEL IT: Small continuous adjustments in the ankle and foot as the balance system works to maintain the position. This is the system learning.

SAFETY:
Have the chair within immediate reach. A timed balance hold should never be more important than safety. Touch down if needed and begin the count again.

Balance Builder 3: Hip Circle Stand

Trains the hip stabilizers through slow rotational movement from a standing position, the same hip control required for the Wave Step and lateral weight transfers.

Starting Position:

Stand with feet slightly wider than hip-width, hands on hips. Chair within reach.

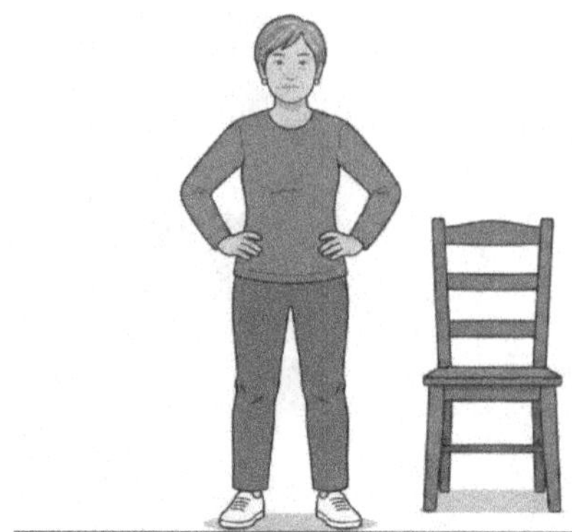

Steps:

1. Begin rotating the hips in a slow horizontal circle, as if drawing a circle with the center of the pelvis. Movement comes from the hips, not the shoulders.

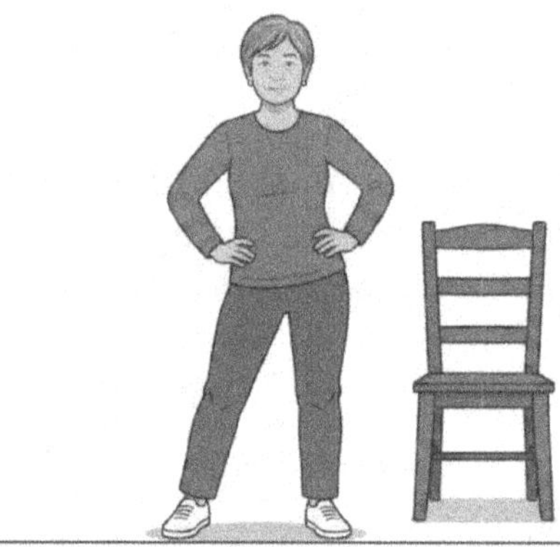

2. Complete five full circles in one direction. Slow and deliberate.

3. Pause for one breath in the center position.

4. Reverse direction for five circles.

BREATHING: Breathe naturally throughout. If you notice breath-holding, exhale completely and restart the breath.

FEEL IT: A loosening in the hip joints and a warmth along the outer hip and lower back as the stabilizers engage.

Balance Builder 4: Tandem Stand

Challenges the balance system in the narrow-base stance that approximates the single-file position of walking. Develops the fine balance control that prevents sideways sway between steps.

Starting Position:

Stand beside the chair, one hand near the chair back. Place the right foot directly in front of the left foot, heel to toe, as if standing on a narrow beam.

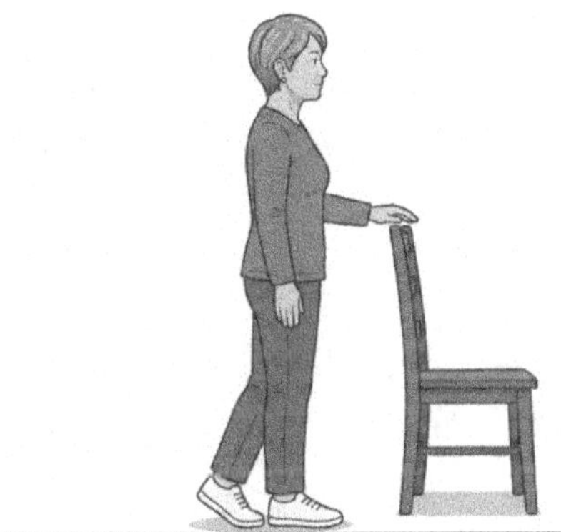

Steps:

1. Release the chair and hold the tandem position. Maintain it for up to 15 seconds.

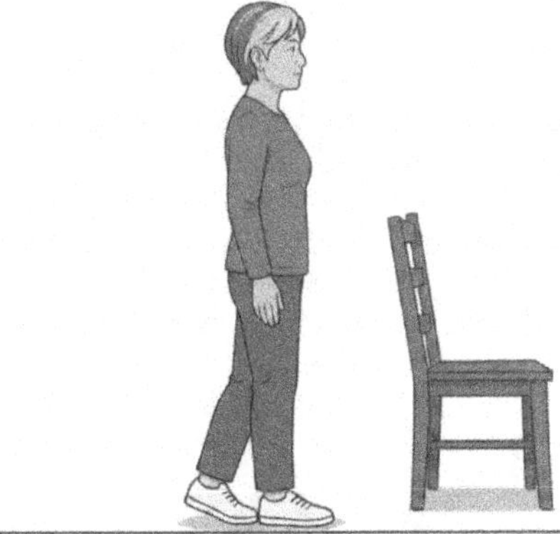

2. If balance fails, touch the chair and begin again.
3. Switch feet: left foot forward, right foot behind. Hold for up to 15 seconds.

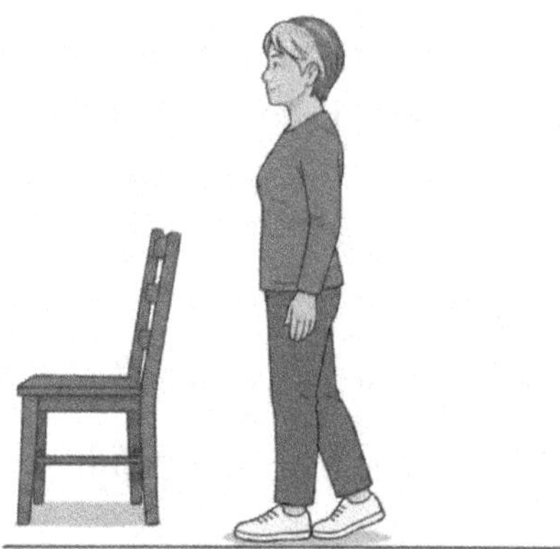

4. Complete two holds on each foot arrangement, building toward 30-second holds over the program.

BREATHING: Slow deliberate breathing throughout. The breath supports the balance.

FEEL IT: More demand than an ordinary standing balance. Small continuous adjustments throughout the hold. This is normal and desirable.

SAFETY:
The tandem stand is the most balance-demanding exercise in this chapter. Always have the chair within immediate reach. Build time gradually. Do not attempt this without a support nearby.

A Small Request

If this book made a difference for you, even in a small way, would you consider leaving an honest review on Amazon or through the website you got a hold of this book?

As an independent author, I don't have the marketing budget of large publishing houses. Reviews are how readers discover books like this. Your feedback truly helps this work reach others who may need it.

It only takes two minutes, and your honest thoughts, positive or critical are genuinely appreciated.

You can leave your review on Amazon by searching the title ***Tai Chi Walking for Weight Loss by Jing Weston*** on Amazon. It takes two minutes, and it matters more than you know.

Chapter 5

The 28-Day Walking Program

This is the operational program. Each day is laid out in full: what to walk, how long, what to focus on. Read the coaching note before each session. It is not decorative. It changes the quality of what follows.

A few things before Day 1. Consistency matters more than perfection. A session where the mechanics were imperfect and you finished counts fully. A session you skip because you expected to do it perfectly does not count at all. On difficult days, use the low-energy option in the Session At a Glance box. Three minutes of the Foundational Breath is still a practice day.

The Safety Reminder in each day's entry is specific to that session's techniques and demands. Read it. It takes five seconds and it is the sentence most likely to prevent the most common problem of that particular day.

Week One – Find Your Footing

This week introduces two techniques: the Rooted Step and the Tai Chi Pace. Nothing else. The sessions are ten minutes long and are done indoors on a clear, flat surface. Week One is not about covering distance or achieving a particular level of performance. It is about making the practice daily and learning what deliberate slow walking actually feels like compared to ordinary walking.

Most people find the Tai Chi Pace uncomfortable in the first two sessions. Not physically uncomfortable. Mentally uncomfortable: the pace feels absurdly slow, the steps feel over-deliberate, and the whole experience feels artificially constructed. This is normal and it passes. By Day 3 the pace begins to feel less odd. By Day 5 it begins to feel useful. Stay with it.

What You Might Feel This Week

• The slow pace may feel unnatural or even slightly frustrating in the first two sessions. This is correct. The discomfort signals that the nervous system is being asked to do something it does not do automatically.

• Mild fatigue in the quadriceps and calf muscles after the first two or three sessions. The sustained slow-loading of each step asks more of these muscles than ordinary walking pace.

• A quiet settling sensation at the end of each session, particularly after the Closing Walk. This is the parasympathetic activation working.

Your Win This Week: Complete a full session every practice day, regardless of how the mechanics feel.

Day 1 – Your First Walk

SESSION AT A GLANCE

Duration: 10 minutes

Techniques: Rooted Step, Tai Chi Pace

Distance: indoor walking path, length of your space

Low-energy option: Foundational Breath practice seated, 3 minutes

---

Jing's Note: *This is the first session. The mechanics will be imprecise and that is expected. Your one job today is to finish. Complete the Pre-Walk Body Check, walk the session at the Tai Chi Pace using the Rooted Step, and close with the Closing Walk. Nothing else is required of Day 1.*

NOTICE TODAY: As the right heel lands, notice whether you feel the surface under the heel or whether the weight transfers too quickly to feel anything. That heel moment is what today's session is training.

SAFETY REMINDER: Ensure your walking path is clear of obstacles before beginning. Check the floor surface at the transition points.

Day 2 – Finding the Heel

SESSION AT A GLANCE

Duration: 10 minutes

Techniques: Rooted Step, Tai Chi Pace

Focus: the pause after heel landing
Low-energy option: Foundational Breath, 3 minutes

Jing's Note: *The heel pause from the Rooted Step is the most important single moment in this program. Today, practice pausing for one full count with the heel down and the toes raised before the weight transfers. If the pause is not happening, slow the pace further until it does.*

NOTICE TODAY: Which foot feels easier to land precisely on the heel? Most people have one side that needs more work. Note which one.

SAFETY REMINDER: Walk only in your cleared indoor space today. Day 2 is not the time to test the mechanics on unfamiliar terrain.

Day 3 – The Roll-Through

SESSION AT A GLANCE
Duration: 10 minutes
Techniques: Rooted Step, Tai Chi Pace
Focus: the heel-to-toe roll within each step
Low-energy option: standing heel raises, 3 minutes

Jing's Note: *Today the focus moves from the heel contact to the roll through the foot: heel, arch, ball, toes. You have been practicing the heel landing. Now add attention to what happens after. The roll-through should feel like a wave moving forward through the foot rather than a flat landing.*

NOTICE TODAY: Can you feel the arch of the foot as the weight passes through it? That brief arch engagement is part of what provides the proprioceptive reading of the surface.

SAFETY REMINDER: If the roll-through produces a sharp sensation in the arch or the ball of the foot, reduce the pace further and consult your footwear fit.

Day 4 – Rest

REST DAY
No formal walking session today. The rest is part of the program.

> **Jing's Note:** *The legs have been asked to do something they did not do before. The muscle adaptation that follows this kind of practice happens during rest, not during effort. Today the rest is as productive as the walking. A gentle walk to the kitchen or the mailbox is fine. A structured walking session is not needed.*

Day 5 – Back to the Path

SESSION AT A GLANCE
Duration: 10 minutes
Techniques: Rooted Step, Tai Chi Pace
Focus: noticing what is different after the rest day
Low-energy option: Foundational Breath, 3 minutes

> **Jing's Note:** *Most people find that the session after a rest day feels more settled than the session before it. The nervous system has had time to consolidate the new patterns. Pay attention to whether the heel pause feels more natural today than it did on Day 3. It usually does.*

NOTICE TODAY: Does the Tai Chi Pace feel slightly less uncomfortable today than it did on Day 1 or 2? Any change at all is significant.

SAFETY REMINDER: Do the Pre-Walk Body Check even on the return-from-rest day. It is especially useful after inactivity, when stiffness may be slightly more pronounced.

Day 6 – Arms Begin

SESSION AT A GLANCE
Duration: 10 minutes
Techniques: Rooted Step, Tai Chi Pace, first introduction to arm swing
Focus: adding gentle arm opposition to the walk
Low-energy option: Foundational Breath, 3 minutes

> **Jing's Note:** *Today add the arm swing from the Tai Chi Pace technique: right arm forward as the left foot steps, left arm forward as the right foot steps. The swing is small and relaxed. If adding the arms disrupts the foot mechanics, drop the arms and restore the feet first. The arms come back when the feet are secure.*

NOTICE TODAY: When both the arm swing and the heel-toe mechanics are working together, does the walk feel any different in the upper body? Some people notice a release of shoulder tension when the arms engage.

SAFETY REMINDER: The arm swing changes the balance slightly. Walk close to your practice support in case the coordination adjustment affects stability.

Day 7 – Rest

REST DAY
No formal walking session today. The rest is part of the program.

Jing's Note: *The legs have been asked to do something they did not do before. The muscle adaptation that follows this kind of practice happens during rest, not during effort. Today the rest is as productive as the walking. A gentle walk to the kitchen or the mailbox is fine. A structured walking session is not needed.*

Slow Is the Point – Understanding Why

Pace should not increase once the mechanics feel settled. The cortisol regulation, fat oxidation, and neural adaptation that make this program effective all depend on maintaining the slow Tai Chi Pace. Speed works against all three goals. If the mechanics feel secure, increase precision rather than distance.

What Counts as a Rest Day

This week includes two rest days: Day 4 and Day 7. Rest days mean no structured walking session, no makeup sessions, and no doubling up, not complete inactivity. A short ordinary walk, gentle stretching, or sitting quietly are all fine. A rest day is not a catch-up day. Do not compress two sessions into one if a session was missed. Daily practice is the design; compressing it reduces the benefit.

Week Two – Lengthen and Steady

Week Two adds Cloud Hands Walking and Wave Step to the sequence. The sessions increase slightly to ten to twelve minutes, and the sequence now runs from the Rooted Step through four techniques before the Closing Walk. The additional length should feel gradual, not demanding. If it feels demanding, the pace is still too fast.

This week the coordination between the arm movements and the leg mechanics is the main technical work. Cloud Hands Walking in particular asks the upper and lower body to do different rhythmic things simultaneously, and that takes a few sessions to settle. Do not expect it to be smooth on Day 8. Expect it to be smooth by Day 12.

What You Might Feel This Week
• The two new techniques may produce a return of the awkwardness from Day 1. This is normal. New mechanics feel unfamiliar before they feel natural.
• An increasing awareness of the walk outside of formal sessions. Some people notice themselves placing their heels more deliberately when walking to the car or down the hallway. This carry-over is the program working.
• The Wave Step will likely produce noticeable fatigue in the outer hip after the first two sessions. That is the hip stabilizer engaging for the first time in a deliberate way.

Your Win This Week: Complete a full session with all four techniques flowing without stopping between them.

Day 8 – Two New Techniques

SESSION AT A GLANCE
Duration: 10-12 minutes
Techniques: Rooted Step, Tai Chi Pace, Cloud Hands Walking, Wave Step
Focus: learning Cloud Hands Walking before adding Wave Step
Low-energy option: Foundational Breath and Rooted Step only, 5 minutes

Jing's Note: *Two new techniques today. Learn Cloud Hands Walking first, practice it for three to four minutes, then practice Wave Step separately. Do not attempt to link all four techniques in sequence on Day 8. The session today is about learning, not flowing.*

NOTICE TODAY: During Cloud Hands Walking, does the upper body turn slightly to follow the arm sweep, or do the arms move independently while the torso stays flat? The turning is what you are looking for.

SAFETY REMINDER: Cloud Hands Walking changes the gaze direction slightly as the eyes follow the arm arc. Ensure the walking path ahead is clear before the gaze moves.

Day 9 – Practicing the Wave

SESSION AT A GLANCE
Duration: 10-12 minutes
Techniques: Rooted Step, Tai Chi Pace, Cloud Hands Walking, Wave Step
Focus: Wave Step hip stability
Low-energy option: Rooted Step and Foundational Breath, 5 minutes

Jing's Note: *Wave Step is the technique most people find most challenging in Week Two because it asks the hip to do something specific that most people's daily walking has not asked of them in years. If the hips are dropping during the lateral step, reduce the step width until the hips can hold level.*

NOTICE TODAY: During the Wave Step, is the transition from the outward step to the closing step smooth, or is there a moment of uncertainty? That transition is where most of the stability work is happening.

SAFETY REMINDER: Do the Wave Step close to the chair in the first two sessions. The lateral movement is more demanding than forward walking.

Day 10 – Linking the Four

SESSION AT A GLANCE
Duration: 10-12 minutes
Techniques: All four in sequence
Focus: transition between techniques
Low-energy option: Rooted Step and Tai Chi Pace, 5 minutes

Jing's Note: *Today attempt to link all four techniques in sequence: Rooted Step into Tai Chi Pace into Cloud Hands Walking into Wave Step into Closing Walk. The transitions between them are the practice. If the transition from one to the next causes a disruption in pace or mechanics, slow down further.*

NOTICE TODAY: Which transition feels least smooth? That is tomorrow's focus.

SAFETY REMINDER: When transitioning from Cloud Hands Walking back to the Rooted Step or Wave Step, return the arms to neutral before beginning the new technique.

Day 11 – Rest

REST DAY
No formal walking session today. The rest is part of the program.

Jing's Note: *The legs have been asked to do something they did not do before. The muscle adaptation that follows this kind of practice happens during rest, not during effort. Today the rest is as productive as the walking. A gentle walk to the kitchen or the mailbox is fine. A structured walking session is not needed.*

Day 12 – Continuous Sequence

SESSION AT A GLANCE
Duration: 10-12 minutes
Techniques: All four continuously
Focus: no pausing between techniques
Low-energy option: Rooted Step, 5 minutes

Jing's Note: *Today the goal is to move through all four techniques without stopping between them. Use the breath as the connector: as one technique ends, the next begins on the next inhale. If you lose your place in the sequence, return to the Rooted Step and continue from there.*

NOTICE TODAY: How far through the continuous sequence does the flow hold before something breaks the continuity? Note the point where it breaks.

SAFETY REMINDER: Continuous walking without stopping requires that the path ahead is clear for the full session duration. Check before beginning.

Day 13 – Quality Check

SESSION AT A GLANCE
Duration: 10-12 minutes
Techniques: All four in sequence
Focus: quality of the heel pause specifically
Low-energy option: Foundational Breath and Rooted Step, 5 minutes

Jing's Note: *Return today to the Rooted Step heel pause and assess its quality after a week of practice. On Day 1, it was a conscious effort. Today, is it beginning to happen automatically? Any reduction in conscious effort required is a sign of neural integration.*

NOTICE TODAY: Compared to Day 1, what is different about how the Rooted Step feels in the body today?

SAFETY REMINDER: The quality check is an assessment, not a performance. Walk at the same pace and with the same caution as every other session.

PROGRESS CHECK

Two weeks of practice. Answer these questions honestly and record the answers next to your Chapter Three baselines.

Does the heel pause in the Rooted Step happen automatically, or do you still consciously produce it? □ Automatic □ Still conscious □ Somewhere between

Does the Tai Chi Pace feel less effortful to maintain than it did in Week One? □ Yes □ About the same □ Variable

Has morning stiffness in the legs changed since Day 1? □ Resolves faster □ About the same □ Variable day to day

Has your awareness of heel placement in ordinary daily walking changed? □ Yes, I notice it more □ Not yet □ Occasionally

Do you feel more confident making the lateral weight shift in the Wave Step than you did on Day 8? □ Yes □ Somewhat □ Still building

Week Three adds the Gathering Walk and the Closing Walk as formal techniques, brings in all six techniques in sequence, and introduces the Balance Builders. Sessions increase to twelve to fifteen minutes. Indoor or outdoor practice both become options. The program begins to feel like something that belongs to you rather than something you are following.

Day 14 – Rest

REST DAY

No formal walking session today. The rest is part of the program.

Jing's Note: *The legs have been asked to do something they did not do before. The muscle adaptation that follows this kind of practice happens during rest, not during effort. Today the rest is as productive as the walking. A gentle walk to the kitchen or the mailbox is fine. A structured walking session is not needed.*

Increasing Distance Without Increasing Risk

Week Two increases technique complexity and session duration, not walking distance. Managing a new technique at the same pace requires more attention and more muscular effort than a familiar one. If sessions feel more demanding than Week One at the same duration, that is the new techniques asking correctly. Keep the pace at or below the Tai Chi Pace throughout.

Week Three – Slim and Strengthen

Week Three completes the six-technique sequence and adds the Balance Builders at the end of each session. Session duration increases to twelve to fifteen minutes. Indoor and outdoor walking are both options from Day 15 onward, with the guidance that outdoor walking should begin on flat, familiar, predictable surfaces before moving to terrain with variation.

This is the week where the fat loss mechanism described in Chapter Two shifts into a more consistent operating state. Three weeks of daily cortisol reduction through deliberate breath-coordinated walking, combined with the leg muscle engagement of the full six-technique sequence, creates a compounding metabolic effect. Most people notice the first body composition signals around Day 17 to 19: clothing fitting slightly differently, morning energy slightly more consistent, the walk feeling less like something they are doing to the body and more like something the body is doing willingly.

What You Might Feel This Week

• The full six-technique sequence will likely feel like too much to track all at once in the first two sessions of this week. This is expected. Sequence familiarity builds within two to three sessions.

• The Balance Builders will produce a specific fatigue in the outer hip and calf muscles after the first use. This is the hip stabilizers and ankle muscles being asked for deliberate work. It resolves within two days.

• Some people report a noticeable improvement in the quality of walking outside of formal sessions around Day 18 to 20. The carry-over effect is becoming measurable.

Your Win This Week: Complete the full six-technique sequence plus at least one Balance Builder on every practice day.

Day 15 – Six Techniques

SESSION AT A GLANCE
Duration: 12-15 minutes
Techniques: All six in sequence
Balance Builders: Standing Heel Raise (10 reps)
Low-energy option: Rooted Step and Foundational Breath, 5 minutes

Jing's Note: *Today introduces the Gathering Walk and the Closing Walk as formal techniques within the sequence. Read through both technique blocks in Chapter Four before this session. Gathering Walk comes between Cloud Hands Walking and Wave Step in the sequence today.*

NOTICE TODAY: During the Gathering Walk, does the arm rise on the inhale actually deepen the breath, or does the breath stay shallow? The arm movement should pull the breath in.

SAFETY REMINDER: Six techniques in sequence is more to hold in attention than four. If the increased cognitive demand affects foot placement, reduce to four techniques and add the additional ones when the sequence feels manageable.

Day 16 – Outdoor Option Begins

SESSION AT A GLANCE
Duration: 12-15 minutes
Techniques: All six in sequence
Setting: indoor or flat outdoor surface
Balance Builders: Standing Heel Raise, Single-Leg Stand (3 holds each side)
Low-energy option: Indoor Rooted Step, 5 minutes

Jing's Note: *If outdoor conditions are suitable today, this is the first day outdoor walking is available. Choose a flat, familiar surface. Walk exactly the same techniques at exactly the same pace. The outdoor surface will provide more proprioceptive input through the foot. Notice it.*

NOTICE TODAY: Outdoors, does the ground surface feel different through the foot compared to the indoor practice surface? What does that difference tell you about the ground?

Day 17 – Pace Variation

SESSION AT A GLANCE
Duration: 12-15 minutes
Techniques: All six in sequence
Variation: alternate two minutes at Tai Chi Pace with one minute at a slightly brisker pace
Balance Builders: Heel Raise, Single-Leg Stand
Low-energy option: Rooted Step only, 8 minutes

Jing's Note: *Today introduces pace variation. Within the session, walk two minutes at the Tai Chi Pace, then allow the pace to increase slightly for one minute, then return to the Tai Chi Pace. The contrast between the paces makes the Tai Chi Pace feel more deliberate and makes the brisker pace feel more controlled. Both effects are useful.*

NOTICE TODAY: At the brisker pace, does the heel pause disappear? If it does, that is the key information: the heel pause is the first thing to be sacrificed when pace increases.

Day 18 – Rest

REST DAY
No formal walking session today. The rest is part of the program.

Jing's Note: *The legs have been asked to do something they did not do before. The muscle adaptation that follows this kind of practice happens during rest, not during effort. Today the rest is as productive as the walking. A gentle walk to the kitchen or the mailbox is fine. A structured walking session is not needed.*

Day 19 – Strengthening Focus

SESSION AT A GLANCE
Duration: 12-15 minutes
Techniques: All six in sequence
Balance Builders: All four, 10 reps or 15-second holds each
Low-energy option: Rooted Step and Wave Step, 5 minutes

Jing's Note: *All four Balance Builders appear together for the first time today. Perform them in order at the end of the walking sequence, before the Closing Walk. The full set takes approximately four minutes. Within the session, they follow the Wave Step and come before the Gathering Walk and Closing Walk.*

NOTICE TODAY: After all four Balance Builders, does anything feel different in the legs during the Gathering Walk and Closing Walk that follow them?

SAFETY REMINDER: The Tandem Stand is the most demanding Balance Builder. Always ensure the chair is within immediate reach before beginning the tandem position.

Day 20 – Continuous and Outdoor

SESSION AT A GLANCE
Duration: 12-15 minutes
Techniques: All six continuously
Setting: outdoor preferred if conditions allow
Balance Builders: All four
Low-energy option: Rooted Step indoors, 8 minutes

Jing's Note: *Today's full six-technique continuous sequence, outdoors where possible, is the most demanding session of the program so far. It is also the most representative of the kind of walking this program is designed to build. Take it seriously without rushing it.*

NOTICE TODAY: Outdoors, how does the heel-to-toe transfer feel on a slightly uneven surface compared to a perfectly flat indoor floor? Describe the difference.

SAFETY REMINDER: Outdoors on any surface with variation, slow the pace further. The slower the pace, the more the foot can read the ground before the weight transfers.

PROGRESS CHECK

Three weeks. Return to your Chapter Three baselines. Compare honestly.

Single-leg balance hold: compare to your Chapter Three baseline. □ Longer hold □ About the same □ Varies by side

Morning stiffness rating: compare to your three-day average from before Day 1. □ Lower □ About the same □ Variable

Does the heel pause in the Rooted Step happen automatically and consistently? □ Yes □ Most of the time □ Still building

Has your walking confidence in daily non-session situations changed? □ Yes, noticeably □ Somewhat □ Not yet measurable

Can you walk the full six-technique sequence continuously without stopping? □ Yes □ With one or two pauses □ Still building

Week Four is the final week. It adds no new techniques. Instead, it consolidates everything built over the previous three weeks, introduces outdoor terrain variation, and ends with the Day 28 Independence Audit. The audit is not a final exam. It is the last measurement in a series of measurements that started before Day 1.

Day 21 – Rest

REST DAY

No formal walking session today. The rest is part of the program.

Jing's Note: *The legs have been asked to do something they did not do before. The muscle adaptation that follows this kind of practice happens during rest, not during effort. Today the rest is as productive as the walking. A gentle walk to the kitchen or the mailbox is fine. A structured walking session is not needed.*

Pace Variation – Where the Fat Burn Accelerates

The pace variation introduced on Day 17 becomes a regular feature in Week Four. Alternating the Tai Chi Pace with slightly brisker intervals within the same session creates an interval-like effect without the joint impact of traditional interval training. The body alternates between deep fat oxidation at the slower pace and slightly elevated muscle demand at the brisker pace. Over the course of the session, both systems are exercised. The cumulative effect on fat metabolism is larger than either pace alone would produce.

Leg and Hip Strength – Feeling It Build

By the end of Week Three, most people can feel the hip stabilizers working during the Wave Step in a way they could not on Day 8. This is not just fitness. It is specific neural recruitment of a muscle group that had been functionally underused. The practical consequence is a pelvis that stays level during the single-leg phases of walking, which reduces the sideways drift that contributes to falls on uneven ground. The measurement is in the walks that become manageable. In the routes that return.

Week Four – Walk With Ownership

Week Four adds no new techniques. It extends what has been built: all six techniques, all four Balance Builders, sessions of fifteen minutes, and where conditions allow, outdoor terrain with some variation. The program ends on Day 28 with the Independence Audit.

Ownership of the technique means the mechanics no longer require conscious tracking. The heel pause happens. The trunk rotation follows the arm sweep. The breath coordinates with the steps. These are happening because the body has practiced them enough to do them reliably. Week Four is where you walk in that state and extend it to more varied conditions.

What You Might Feel This Week

• The full fifteen-minute session will feel longer than Week Three sessions initially. By Day 25 it will feel natural.

• Some people notice, around Day 24 to 26, that they are walking differently in non-session contexts without consciously deciding to. The gait changes have become default.

• The Independence Audit on Day 28 may reveal changes that are larger or smaller than expected. Both require honest reading. The honest reading is the useful one.

Your Win This Week: Complete every session including the Balance Builders, and walk at least two sessions outdoors on terrain with some variation.

Day 22 – Full Program

SESSION AT A GLANCE
Duration: 15 minutes
Techniques: All six in continuous sequence
Balance Builders: All four

Low-energy option: Rooted Step and Foundational Breath, 5 minutes

Jing's Note: *Fifteen minutes. The longest session of the program. The pace stays the same. The duration extends. Allow the extension to feel natural rather than effortful. If it feels significantly harder than Day 20, check whether the pace has crept upward during the week.*

NOTICE TODAY: At the fifteen-minute mark, what is different about the quality of the walk compared to the first five minutes? Many people notice a settling into the practice that happens only after several minutes.

SAFETY REMINDER: Increase session duration gradually rather than from twelve to fifteen minutes in one jump if the jump feels too large. Twelve minutes for the first two sessions of Week Four is acceptable.

Day 23 – Outdoor Terrain

SESSION AT A GLANCE
Duration: 15 minutes
Techniques: All six in sequence
Setting: outdoor, flat with slight variation
Balance Builders: All four
Low-energy option: Indoor full sequence, 10 minutes

Jing's Note: *Today introduces terrain with slight variation: a sidewalk with a join in the surface, a gentle slope, a textured surface. Walk the full technique sequence on this terrain at the Tai Chi Pace. The variation in the surface will make the heel pause more important and the body's proprioceptive reading more active.*

NOTICE TODAY: On a slightly uneven surface, does the body make automatic small adjustments, or does every irregularity require conscious attention? The degree of automation is the degree of integration.

SAFETY REMINDER: Choose outdoor terrain that is familiar and predictable for Day 23. This is not the session for uneven ground that is new to you.

Day 24 – Rest

> **REST DAY**
> No formal walking session today. The rest is part of the program.

> **Jing's Note:** *The legs have been asked to do something they did not do before. The muscle adaptation that follows this kind of practice happens during rest, not during effort. Today the rest is as productive as the walking. A gentle walk to the kitchen or the mailbox is fine. A structured walking session is not needed.*

Day 25 – Pace Variation Outdoors

> **SESSION AT A GLANCE**
> Duration: 15 minutes
> Techniques: All six in sequence
> Variation: two minutes Tai Chi Pace, one minute slightly brisker, alternating
> Balance Builders: All four
> Low-energy option: Tai Chi Pace only, 10 minutes

> **Jing's Note:** *Today combines the pace variation pattern from Day 17 with outdoor terrain. The brisker pace outdoors is a more honest test of whether the heel mechanics hold under pressure. They will hold better than they did three weeks ago.*

> **NOTICE TODAY:** At the brisker pace outdoors, is the heel pause maintained, reduced, or lost? This is the measure of technique stability under pace pressure.

> **SAFETY REMINDER:** Outdoors, pace variation means the slightly brisker pace remains well below ordinary walking speed. Do not walk at an ordinary pace and call it a brisker interval.

Day 26 – Last Full Session

> **SESSION AT A GLANCE**
> Duration: 15 minutes
> Techniques: All six continuously
> Setting: your choice of indoor or outdoor
> Balance Builders: All four

Low-energy option: Foundational Breath and Rooted Step, 5 minutes

Jing's Note: *The last full walking session before the Independence Audit. Walk it with full attention. The Closing Walk at the end of this session is the last practice close before the program completes.*

NOTICE TODAY: Walk to your usual turning point and stand for a moment before turning back. What is different about how that standing feels now compared to how standing felt before Day 1?

SAFETY REMINDER: Continue the Pre-Walk Body Check even on Day 26. The ritual protects consistency regardless of session number.

Day 27 – Rest

REST DAY
No formal walking session today. The rest is part of the program.

Jing's Note: *The legs have been asked to do something they did not do before. The muscle adaptation that follows this kind of practice happens during rest, not during effort. Today the rest is as productive as the walking. A gentle walk to the kitchen or the mailbox is fine. A structured walking session is not needed.*

Day 28 – Independence Audit

SESSION AT A GLANCE
Duration: 15 minutes
Techniques: Full six-technique sequence
Balance Builders: All four
Closing: Day 28 Independence Audit after the session

Jing's Note: *Twenty-eight days. Walk the session. Hold the Closing Walk breath cycles for five full counts rather than three. Let the session land. Then complete the Independence Audit below.*

NOTICE TODAY: Walk this session with your attention on the body rather than on the technique. The techniques are familiar enough now that they can run in the background. Walk and notice what the body is doing.

SAFETY REMINDER: Complete the full Pre-Walk Body Check before this session. Note any changes from the earliest checks.

Outdoor Routes, Uneven Ground, Stairs

By Day 28, most people who have completed the outdoor sessions have encountered uneven terrain, at least one set of steps, and the kinds of surface transitions that were uncomfortable in Week One. The purpose of the outdoor progression in Weeks Three and Four is not to make the program harder. It is to apply the mechanics to real-world conditions before the program ends.

The most common report from participants who complete this program is not improved walking endurance. It is that specific places and situations have changed. The uneven pavement route is back on the list. The parking lot is navigable again. These independence gains are the real measure of what twenty-eight days of deliberate practice has built.

Stairs are where many older adults feel the most acute limitation and are directly addressed by the program's combination of heel mechanics, hip stability, and single-leg balance training. The approach: slow down before the first step, lead with the heel, pause at the top of the transfer, keep the gaze forward. This is the Rooted Step applied vertically.

End of Week Four: Independence Audit

PROGRESS CHECK

This is not a grade. It is the final comparison in a series that began before Day 1 in Chapter Three. Take your time with it. Write the answers next to your original baselines.

Single-leg balance hold: compare to your Chapter Three baseline. □ Significantly longer □ Somewhat longer □ About the same □ Variable

Morning stiffness level: compare to your three-day pre-program average. □ Lower □ Slightly lower □ About the same

Comfortable walking distance: has it changed, and in what direction? □ Greater □ About the same □ Changed in quality rather than distance

Is there a specific route, place, or situation that is more accessible or less anxiety-producing now than before Day 1? □ Yes □ Not yet, but I notice smaller changes □ No change I can identify

Does the heel-to-toe transfer happen automatically in ordinary daily walking? □ Yes, consistently □ Sometimes, when I notice it □ Not yet in daily walking

Whatever the numbers show, the act of completing 28 days of deliberate daily practice is itself a result. The habit is the foundation. Chapter Eight addresses what comes next, how to read the audit honestly, and how to continue building from here regardless of whether the changes were large, modest, or quieter than expected.

Chapter 6

Eating for the Miles

This chapter is not a diet plan. It is a practical account of how food, water, and rest interact with the specific demands of a walking practice for older adults. Small adjustments, aligned with what the body needs for this kind of movement, produce results that larger dietary changes imposed alongside a new exercise program often do not.

Why Walkers Need a Different Approach to Food

Walking is a weight-bearing activity. It asks the legs to support and move the body's full weight with every step, repeatedly, for the duration of the session. The muscles, tendons, and joints doing that work have specific nutritional requirements that a general healthy diet advice framework does not always address. Understanding those requirements changes what you prioritize at the table, not dramatically, but specifically.

The first requirement is adequate protein. After sixty, the body's ability to synthesize muscle protein from dietary protein declines. The same amount of protein that maintained muscle mass at forty-five may be insufficient at sixty-five. For a walking program that is asking the quadriceps, calf muscles, and hip stabilizers to do deliberate work they have not done recently, protein availability at the right times is the difference between those muscles rebuilding and adapting and those muscles producing soreness without improvement.

The practical protein target for an older adult beginning this program is approximately half a gram per pound of body weight per day. For most people in the target age range this is 60 to 80 grams. This is not a large amount and is achievable through ordinary food: two eggs, a cup of Greek yogurt, a palm-sized serving of fish or chicken, and a handful of nuts across three meals will typically meet the target without any calculation. Spreading protein across meals matters as much as the total daily amount, because the body can only synthesize muscle protein from a single meal at a limited rate.

The second food-specific requirement for walkers in this age group is anti-inflammatory nutrition. The heel-to-toe mechanics this program uses, done daily, produce a small but accumulating demand on the ankle and knee joints. Supporting those joints through nutrition reduces the background inflammation that would otherwise build over the first two weeks and can produce enough discomfort to disrupt the program. Anti-inflammatory eating does not require exotic ingredients. It requires consistent use of the foods that are already understood to reduce systemic inflammation.

The relationship between protein adequacy and inflammation is worth noting. When the body does not have sufficient protein available for muscle repair, it draws on muscle tissue as a protein source through a process called catabolism. Catabolism produces inflammatory byproducts that add to the joint inflammation the walking program is already managing through technique and nutrition. Adequate protein is therefore both a direct muscle support measure and an indirect anti-inflammatory measure. Meeting the protein target reduces the catabolism that would otherwise drive the background inflammation upward during the adaptation weeks.

Anti-Inflammatory Eating for Joint-Friendly Movement

The foods that reduce joint inflammation for walkers fall into predictable categories.

Fatty fish.

Salmon, mackerel, sardines, and anchovies provide omega-3 fatty acids that directly reduce prostaglandin-driven joint inflammation. Two to three servings per week is the threshold at which measurable anti-inflammatory effects are documented. Tinned sardines and mackerel are as effective as fresh fish and considerably more accessible for daily eating.

Berries and dark leafy greens.

Blueberries, strawberries, spinach, kale, and broccoli provide polyphenols and antioxidants that reduce oxidative stress in the joints. A handful of berries at breakfast and a serving of leafy greens at one meal covers most of the daily requirement. The specific compounds involved are heat-stable, so cooking the greens does not eliminate their effect.

Olive oil.

Used as the primary cooking fat, olive oil provides oleocanthal, a compound with documented anti-inflammatory properties similar in mechanism to ibuprofen, though significantly less potent. The practical benefit for walkers is that consistent use of olive oil as a cooking fat, rather than occasional use, reduces background inflammation in a way that compounds over weeks.

Whole grains over refined grains.

Refined carbohydrates, white bread, white rice, pastries, sweetened cereals, drive inflammatory processes through their effect on blood sugar and insulin. Whole grain versions of the same foods produce a much slower glucose response and substantially lower inflammatory signaling. The substitution does not require eliminating these foods. It requires choosing the whole grain version as the default.

What to reduce.

Highly processed foods, particularly those with added sugar and refined vegetable oils, are the primary dietary drivers of systemic inflammation for most people. Alcohol, at levels beyond one drink per day, impairs sleep quality significantly and disrupts the overnight muscle protein synthesis that makes the walking practice productive. Neither needs to be eliminated completely. Both need to be genuinely reduced, not nominally reduced, during the program.

What to Eat Before and After Your Walk

The timing of food relative to the walking session matters for two reasons. The first is energy availability: the session requires the legs to do sustained moderate work, and doing that work on a completely empty stomach produces the light-headedness that some older adults experience during the single-leg balance phases. The second is the recovery window: in the two to three hours after the session, the muscles are maximally receptive to protein for repair and adaptation. Missing this window with a low-protein or no-food period reduces the training benefit of the session.

Before the session.

A small snack containing a combination of carbohydrate and protein, consumed thirty to forty-five minutes before the session, provides sufficient fuel without weighing down the digestive system. Half a banana with a tablespoon of almond butter, a small pot of Greek yogurt, or two whole grain crackers with a thin slice of cheese are all suitable. The goal is not a substantial meal. It is enough available fuel to prevent energy dips during the balance-demanding phases of the session.

If you practice in the morning and prefer not to eat before walking, at minimum drink a full glass of water before beginning. Mild dehydration, which is common in older adults on waking, affects balance and cognitive function in ways that are directly relevant to the attention this practice requires.

After the session.

A protein-containing meal or snack within sixty minutes of finishing the session takes advantage of the post-exercise insulin sensitivity window. The muscles are primed to absorb amino acids for repair. Eggs with vegetables, oatmeal with Greek yogurt stirred in and berries on top, a tin of sardines with whole grain crackers and sliced cucumber, or cottage cheese with fruit and walnuts all meet the requirement. Speed of preparation matters: a five-minute meal happens; a thirty-minute meal often does not.

Staying Hydrated on the Move

Dehydration and balance are directly connected. Even mild dehydration, defined as a one to two percent reduction in body water, affects proprioception, reaction time, and cognitive clarity. All three are directly relevant to the quality of walking this program depends on. After sixty, the thirst mechanism becomes less reliable as a hydration signal. Many older adults are mildly dehydrated throughout the day without ever feeling thirsty.

The practical solution is habit-based rather than thirst-based hydration. A glass of water before the Pre-Walk Body Check, and another glass within thirty minutes of finishing the session, provides a reliable minimum baseline. For outdoor sessions in warm weather or when the session produces visible perspiration, a third glass during or after the session is appropriate.

A simple way to assess hydration adequacy is urine color. Pale yellow indicates adequate hydration. Dark yellow or amber indicates mild dehydration that needs addressing before the session begins. This assessment takes two seconds and is more reliable than thirst as a hydration indicator for older adults. Making it a morning habit alongside the Pre-Walk Body

Check requires no additional effort and removes one of the most common but least recognized performance limiters for this population.

Electrolyte balance matters alongside fluid intake for people who walk regularly in warm conditions. Sodium, potassium, and magnesium are lost in sweat, and low levels of any of the three affect muscle function and proprioception. Ordinary food provides sufficient electrolytes for indoor practice and short outdoor sessions in moderate temperatures. For extended outdoor sessions in warm weather, adding a small amount of salt to food or choosing electrolyte-containing fluids becomes more relevant.

Caffeinated drinks, coffee and tea, contribute to fluid intake and do not need to be avoided. Their mild diuretic effect is offset by the water content at normal consumption levels. Alcohol is genuinely dehydrating and disrupts the sleep quality that is as important to this program as the walking itself.

Rest, Recovery, and the Walking Body

Rest days are when the adaptation happens. This is not a motivational statement. It is physiology. During rest, the muscle fibers that were worked during the walking sessions undergo repair. The neural pathways that were trained become more efficient. Hormones involved in muscle protein synthesis, particularly growth hormone, are released primarily during deep sleep. A rest day followed by poor sleep is a rest day that produced less adaptation than a well-slept one.

The rest days in this program are scheduled specifically. They are not days to catch up on missed sessions. They are not days to do a different form of exercise to compensate. They are days for the body to use the work that was done. Gentle walking to destinations, stretching, and ordinary household movement are all fine on rest days. A structured walking session is not appropriate on a scheduled rest day.

Between sessions on practice days, the legs benefit from movement that is different from the formal session: standing, gentle stretching of the calf and quadriceps, walking at an ordinary pace. The formal session is the deliberate practice. The rest of the day's movement supports the session without replacing it.

Calf stretching is particularly useful for walkers over sixty because the calf muscles and Achilles tendon tend to tighten with age and reduced walking range, reducing ankle mobility and making the heel strike harder to execute fully. A simple standing calf stretch against a wall, held for twenty to thirty seconds on each side after the session, maintains the ankle flexibility that the Rooted Step depends on. This takes ninety seconds and addresses one of the most common physical limiters in this population.

Sleep and Gait

The connection between sleep quality and next-day balance is direct and specific enough to be worth stating plainly. A night of poor sleep, particularly a night with reduced deep sleep, produces measurably worse proprioceptive function the following morning. The feet and ankles send less precise signals to the brain about ground contact and position. The brain's integration of those signals is slower. The result is a walking session where the heel pause feels harder to maintain, the single-leg balance phases feel less stable, and the risk of an unexpected stumble is higher than after a well-slept night.

For people beginning this program who are already managing disrupted sleep, the good news is that consistent deliberate walking practice improves sleep quality through the cortisol reduction mechanism described in Chapter Two. The practice and the sleep reinforce each other. Better sleep produces better walking. Better walking produces better sleep. The entry point is the practice, and the sleep improvement follows it, usually within two to three weeks.

The practical sleep guidance for people doing this program is consistent and modest: keep a consistent wake time even on rest days, because the wake time is the strongest regulator of the sleep-wake cycle. Avoid screen use in the forty-five minutes before bed, because the light exposure delays the onset of melatonin and delays sleep. Practice the Closing Walk breath pattern, or simply the Foundational Breath, in the minutes before sleep. The parasympathetic activation it produces supports sleep onset in the same way it closes the walking session. A cooler bedroom temperature, around 65 to 68 degrees Fahrenheit, supports the drop in core body temperature that initiates deep sleep. These are not complicated interventions. They are specific adjustments that compound over weeks into meaningfully better sleep quality.

Chapter 7

Rebuilding Independence Step by Step

Independence is a plain word for something that is not plain at all when you start to lose it. This chapter is about what the walking practice in this book actually builds toward, and what it gives back.

The Real Goal – Walking Life, Not Just Exercise

The 28-day program is an exercise program. But the goal was never the program. The goal is what the program produces in the hours, days, and months that follow it: a body that can be relied upon to do the things that daily life requires.

What independence actually means for an older adult who has been gradually restricting their movement is specific and physical. It means walking to the mailbox without wondering whether you will manage the return journey. It means crossing a parking lot from the far end because that was the only space, without the low-grade anxiety that used to accompany that situation. It means saying yes to an invitation that involves walking on unfamiliar ground because the unfamiliar ground is no longer the deciding factor.

These are small things. People who have them take them completely for granted. People who have lost them, or are in the process of losing them, know exactly what they are worth. Jing Weston has sat beside many people over the years who gave up a particular place or a particular activity not in one decisive moment but through a series of quiet withdrawals, each individually sensible, accumulating into a significantly narrowed life. What they wanted was not a fitness program. They wanted those places and those activities back. The program is the mechanism. Independence is the goal.

The social dimension of independence is as significant as the physical one. Many older adults find that reduced walking confidence leads to a reduction in social participation that is separate from any explicit decision to withdraw. They simply do not go to places that feel uncertain, and over time those places come to include more and more of the locations where social activity happens. Rebuilding walking confidence does not automatically rebuild social participation, but it removes the physical obstacle that was preventing it. The rest is a choice. Having the choice is the point.

The practice this book teaches is specifically calibrated to rebuild the physical capacities that make independence possible: reliable heel-to-toe weight transfer, confident single-leg balance, responsive hip stabilizers, and the proprioceptive reading of ground surfaces. These are not abstract fitness qualities. They are the mechanics of every specific act of independence described above.

The emotional experience of genuinely rebuilding independence is not uniform. Some people find that the physical improvements happen faster than the psychological adjustment to them. They have better balance and a more reliable gait, but they continue to make cautious choices out of habit. The habit of caution, built over months or years of genuine physical limitation, does not dissolve automatically when the physical limitation improves. It needs to be deliberately tested, with the same graduated approach the program used for the balance exercises. Small tests, in safe and familiar environments, that confirm what the body can now do.

Stairs, Slopes, and Uneven Ground With Confidence

Stairs are the most common physical barrier that older adults with walking confidence problems name. The approach this program builds handles stairs directly: slow down before the first step, lead with the heel, pause briefly at the top of the transfer before committing the body's weight to the new level, keep the gaze forward rather than looking down at the step. Handrails are appropriate and sensible. Using a handrail is not a defeat. It is a tool, exactly as the chair was a tool in the balance exercises.

Slopes require a modification of the Rooted Step mechanics. On a downhill slope, the heel lands but the weight transfer must be slower because gravity is helping it happen faster than is safe. Consciously resisting the pull of the slope during the transfer, engaging the quadriceps to brake rather than allowing gravity to pull the body forward, is the specific skill that prevents downhill stumbles. The deliberate braking movement that the program builds through three weeks of slow weight transfers is exactly the right preparation for slopes.

On an uphill slope, the heel strike remains but the push-off from the rear foot becomes more important. The calf muscles and the gluteal muscles do more work than on flat ground. By

Week Three of the program, these muscles have been specifically trained through the Heel Raise balance builder and the daily Rooted Step practice. The uphill walk will be more demanding. It will not be as threatening as it might have been before Day 1.

Uneven ground, the cracked sidewalk, the packed gravel, the grass between the car and the entrance, requires the proprioceptive reading that the program has been training since Day 1. The foot that reads the ground before committing the body's weight has a moment to register irregularity and send the adjustment signal before the fall risk materializes. The foot that flat-lands at ordinary walking speed does not have that moment. After twenty-eight days of deliberate heel-pause practice, the reading happens. Not perfectly, not always, but more reliably than before.

Grocery Runs, Errands, and Getting Out Again

The practical test of this program's success is not a balance measurement in a doctor's office. It is whether the person who completed it went to more places in the week after Day 28 than in the week before Day 1. Whether they walked to the shops rather than drove. Whether they took the longer route because they chose to rather than the shorter one because they had to.

Grocery runs deserve specific mention because they involve a combination of demands that make them disproportionately challenging: a shopping trolley or basket to manage, a crowded and unpredictable aisle environment, floor surfaces that change from entrance to produce section to refrigerated section, and the need to stop, pivot, reach, and turn while carrying weight. These are real demands. The program addresses each of them. The pivot turn practiced in the technique blocks. The lateral weight shift from the Wave Step. The single-leg balance from the balance builders. The carry is not specifically trained, but the stability that makes carrying safer is.

Errands and social outings involve an element that is harder to train directly: the willingness to go. The fear-tension cycle described in Chapter One narrows the social world as much as the physical one. People stop accepting invitations to places they are not certain they can navigate without difficulty. The confidence that comes from competence, from having practiced the specific mechanics that make navigation possible, does not just change the physical experience. It changes the calculation. More invitations get a yes.

The carry is worth addressing specifically. Carrying a shopping bag, a bag, a grandchild, anything that shifts the body's center of gravity, changes the balance demand of walking significantly. A bag carried in one hand creates an asymmetric load that the hip stabilizers must compensate for. After three weeks of deliberate hip stabilizer work through the Wave Step and the balance builders, this compensation is more reliable than before. The walk with a full shopping bag is not the same as the walk without one. But it is more manageable than it was before Day 1.

When to Walk With Support

Walking with support, a cane, a walking frame, a companion's arm, is appropriate and sensible for people whose balance is not yet safe without it. This program does not ask anyone to abandon support before they are ready. The chair-assisted modifications in every technique block are there precisely because some people need support while they are building the capacity that will eventually allow unsupported practice.

People who use walking aids frequently ask when they will no longer need them. The honest answer is that some people will always use a cane for certain conditions, such as highly uneven terrain or crowded environments, even after their everyday walking balance has substantially improved. The aim is not to eliminate the walking aid entirely in all conditions. It is to reduce the range of conditions that require it, so that the cane or frame is a tool for specific situations rather than a constant companion for all walking.

The progression from supported to unsupported walking is not a goal with a deadline. It happens when it happens, and it happens through the same mechanism as every other capacity this program builds: repetition of the specific movement with slightly less support at each stage. If you are using a cane at the start of the program, the progression might be: cane throughout Week One, cane for outdoor sessions and chair for indoor sessions in Week Two, chair only for the balance builders in Week Three, unsupported for the walking techniques in Week Four. Or it might take longer. The timeline is not the point.

What matters is that the direction of travel is toward less support, even if the steps are small and the pace is slow. A person who needs a cane in Week One and uses it with less reliance by Day 28 has made real progress, even if they still need the cane. A person who needs a cane in Week One and uses it with the same reliance by Day 28 has used this program to maintain their current capacity, which is also a genuine outcome worth acknowledging.

The Long Walk

What consistent deliberate movement gives back over years is not a return to some earlier physical state. The body at seventy is not the body at fifty, and the practice is not pretending otherwise. What it gives back is proportion: the capacity the body has at any given age, used as fully as that age allows.

Jing Weston has worked with people in their eighties who began deliberate walking practice after years of increasing restriction and who, at eighty-three or eighty-five, were walking more confidently than they had at seventy-eight. Not more distance. Not faster. More confidently. The mechanics were more reliable. The heel pause was happening. The hip stabilizers were providing the level pelvis that makes each step more precise. The walk to the shops was not a negotiation. It was a walk.

That is the long walk. Not the distance. The quality of the step, maintained or rebuilt, for as many years as the practice continues. It is available to anyone willing to spend ten minutes each morning and pay attention to how they move. That is the full requirement, and it has always been the full requirement. Everything else follows from it. This book gave you the ten minutes. The long walk is what you do with them.

Chapter 8

After Day 28

The program is finished. Before you decide what happens next, read this chapter. It will help you interpret what the Independence Audit shows and give you a clear picture of what comes from here.

Your Independence Audit – What's Actually Changed

The Independence Audit at the end of Day 28 asks you to compare five specific measures to the baselines you established before Day 1. The comparison is the most honest account available of what twenty-eight days of deliberate walking practice has done in your body. But reading it honestly requires understanding what the measures can and cannot tell you.

If your single-leg balance hold is significantly longer on Day 28 than it was in Chapter Three, that is a structural change in the hip stabilizer and ankle muscle capacity, and in the neural pathways that manage single-leg balance. That change does not disappear when the program ends. It is built into the body now, and it will persist as long as practice continues.

If your morning stiffness rating has decreased, that is the synovial fluid and circulation effects of daily movement compounding over four weeks. The joints that receive daily deliberate loading produce more lubricating fluid and maintain better circulation than joints that are only moved at ordinary walking pace. That improvement will also persist with continued practice, and will likely continue to improve over the following months.

If the heel pause is now happening automatically in ordinary daily walking, that is the most significant neural integration the program produces. It means the nervous system has incorporated the new pattern into its default gait program. Falls that happen from flat-footed gait on unexpected surfaces are less likely, because the foot is now reading the surface before committing weight to it. This change is the one with the most direct and specific fall prevention consequence.

If the audit shows that a specific route, place, or situation is more accessible than before Day 1, that is the independence goal achieved at a concrete and specific level. It is worth naming that thing explicitly, writing it down, and holding it as the measure of what the program did. Not the balance numbers. The place that is accessible again.

When Progress Was Clear

Clear progress in all five audit measures after twenty-eight days is the best possible outcome and is also genuinely common for people who completed the program consistently. If this is your result, the decision that matters most is not what to do next but what to protect. The progress you have made is not permanent without continued practice. It is the product of daily repetition over four weeks, and it will be maintained by daily repetition beyond those four weeks.

The simplest continuation is to run the program again from Week One. The experience of the second run is qualitatively different from the first: the techniques are familiar, the pace settles more quickly, the coaching notes in Chapter Five read differently when the mechanics they refer to are already established. Most people find the second run produces a deeper integration of the same improvements rather than entirely new ones.

An alternative for people who do not want to follow the structured program a second time is to build their own daily practice from Chapter Four. Use the six techniques as a library: choose the ones that address the session's particular intention for that day. A balance-focused day might emphasize the Wave Step and the Balance Builders. A circulation day might emphasize the Gathering Walk and Cloud Hands Walking at a slightly brisker pace. The program taught the techniques. Using them freely is the next stage.

When Progress Was Quiet

Quiet progress means the audit numbers have not changed dramatically, but something is different in ways the specific measures do not capture. The walk feels different from the inside. The heel pause is more reliable. The gait on familiar terrain feels slightly more settled, even if the balance hold time on a single-leg test has not extended significantly. These are real changes and they are worth taking seriously rather than dismissing because they do not show up as a number.

Quiet progress after a complete twenty-eight-day program is usually the result of one of three things. Inconsistent sessions, where the daily repetition that produces neural adaptation was not quite daily enough to produce the full adaptation within four weeks. This resolves with a second program run at higher completion rate. Insufficient sleep, where the overnight consolidation of the neural patterns trained during sessions was disrupted by poor sleep quality. The connection between sleep and gait adaptation is specific and direct: without adequate deep sleep, the neural consolidation that makes the walking improvements permanent does not happen at full capacity. And baseline physical condition significantly below the program's assumptions, where the starting point was so deconditioned that four weeks was not sufficient to produce dramatic measured changes, though real changes are nonetheless occurring beneath the surface.

In any of these cases, the appropriate response is to continue, not to stop. The changes are slower than ideal but they are happening. A second program run, or a continued daily practice using the Chapter Four library, will build on what the first twenty-eight days started.

How to Handle Setbacks Without Losing Ground

Setbacks in a walking program take several forms: illness that prevents walking for a week or more, a pain flare in a hip or knee, weather that makes outdoor practice impossible for an extended period, or a disruption to the daily routine that breaks the practice habit. Each requires a specific response rather than a general one.

Illness. Do not walk through illness that produces fever, significant fatigue, or any respiratory symptoms. Wait until you are recovered and then return at the beginning of Week One, not at whatever week you left. The body that recovers from illness needs to rebuild its capacity the same way the body at the start of the program did. Starting from Week One after illness is not a failure. It is appropriate periodization.

Pain flare. A pain flare in a hip or knee during the program requires reducing to the chair-assisted modifications and the low-impact techniques until the flare resolves. The Foundational Breath and the Wave Step lateral weight transfer can both be done from a chair. The balance builders can be done with full chair support. The practice continues in a reduced form, which maintains the habit and preserves as much of the adaptation as the pain allows.

Habit disruption. Travel, family demands, schedule changes, all disrupt exercise habits. The response that maintains the most ground is doing a shortened session, five minutes of the Rooted Step at the Tai Chi Pace, rather than skipping entirely. A shortened session is a practice day. It keeps the habit intact. Skipping is not a practice day, and re-establishing the habit after a break is harder than maintaining it through a reduced-form session. If the environment does not permit even five minutes of walking, the Foundational Breath practice done standing still is a practice day in the minimal sense: the habit signals persists even when the walking cannot.

Designing Your Own Walking Life From Here

The goal of this program was never to make you dependent on it. It was to give you a body that moves more reliably and a practice that supports it. What you do with that from Day 29 onward is genuinely open.

The minimum effective maintenance practice is ten minutes of the Rooted Step and the Tai Chi Pace daily, with the Closing Walk at the end of each session. This is sufficient to maintain the neural and muscular adaptations the program built. It requires nothing that was not already part of the practice. It is the irreducible core.

Maintenance is not the ceiling. It is the floor. What the minimum practice maintains, a longer or more varied practice builds upon. The neural adaptation to a new movement pattern continues to refine for months after the initial learning phase. A person who is still practicing the Rooted Step six months after Day 28 is walking with a heel-to-toe pattern that is more automatic, more reliable, and more transferable to novel terrain than the one they had on Day 28 itself. The improvements do not plateau at the end of the program. They plateau when the practice stops.

Extensions are possible in any direction. More session time, up to thirty minutes, produces proportionally larger cardiovascular and metabolic benefits without qualitatively changing the practice. Additional outdoor routes, including more challenging terrain, build on the base the program established. Introducing new walking environments, urban streets, parks, shopping precincts, applies the mechanics to the real-world conditions independence requires. None of these extensions require new instruction. They require the same practice applied to new contexts.

The walking life you build from here is yours and it belongs entirely to you. The program gave you the techniques and the habit. The independence is what you do with them.

Did You Find This Book Quite Helpful?

If it did, then that's worth something and deserves a place on Amazon.

A short review on Amazon takes two minutes and costs nothing. But for an independent author with no marketing budget, it means everything. It is how the next reader finds this book. It is how a daughter finds the right gift for her aging mother and father. It is how this work continues to reach the people it was made for.

Search ***Tai Chi Walking for Weight Loss by Jing Weston*** on Amazon. One or two honest sentences is all it takes.

Thank you for reading. It was an honor to take this trip with you.

Conclusion

What 28 Days of Showing Up Built

The 28-day program built something that does not exist in the body before the practice begins. Not fitness in the general sense. A specific neural pattern: the heel contacts the ground, the foot reads the surface, the body waits for the reading before the weight transfers. That moment, which takes less than a second and which most people's gait does not contain, is what the program spent twenty-eight sessions installing.

It is also what prevents the specific category of falls that happen from flat-footed gait on unexpected surfaces. Not all falls. Not all of the time. But a measurable proportion of the falls that happen to people who do not practice deliberate heel-to-toe walking and who encounter uneven ground at ordinary walking speed. Twenty-eight days of showing up did that.

The other thing the program built is a daily practice. The habit of ten minutes each morning with specific attention on how the body moves. This is more durable than any specific fitness improvement, because the fitness improvement is produced by the practice and continues to be produced as long as the practice continues. The habit is the mechanism. The independence is the output.

The Walker You Were, the Walker You Are Now

Whatever brought you to this book, there was a version of you before Day 1 who was walking in a particular way, with a particular degree of confidence or caution, to a particular range of places and situations. That is the baseline the Chapter Three assessment captured.

The walker you are now, having completed twenty-eight sessions of deliberate practice, is different in at least some of those dimensions. The difference might be dramatic or quiet. It might show up as a number on a balance test or as a place you went this week that you would not have gone to before. Both are real. Both count. The measure that matters most is the one that is most specific to your own life: the route you walked, the errand you did, the invitation you said yes to.

Walking is not a performance. It is not a competitive activity. It is the means by which a person moves through the world and participates in their own life. Anything that makes the walking more reliable makes the participation more reliable. That is what this program was always about.

A Final Word from the Author

I have watched many people start this kind of practice. The ones who stay with it longest are not the ones who start with the greatest physical capacity. They are the ones who start with a genuine reason to keep going.

For most of the people I have worked with, the reason is specific. Not abstract health. Not general fitness. A specific place they wanted to get back to. A specific situation they wanted to manage without fear. A specific person they wanted to keep up with. Those reasons are more durable than willpower. When the ten minutes feels inconvenient, the specific reason is still there.

Find your reason if you have not already. Hold it specifically, not vaguely. The walk to the mailbox. The parking lot at the end of the road. The steps outside a friend's house. The specific real thing that a more reliable walking body makes possible. That is what you are practicing toward.

Every step you take with intention is practice. Every heel that lands and reads the ground before the weight follows is practice. Every breath that coordinates with the movement is practice. This does not require twenty-eight days or a formal program or a scheduled session. It requires the habit of paying attention to how you move. You have been building that habit. Keep it.

The practice is yours now. Go walk.

About the Author

Jing Weston has practiced Tai Chi for more than two decades and has spent most of that time working with older adults, people managing chronic conditions, and beginners who came to movement late and found it transformed how they lived. He began with group classes at a community center and eventually worked one-on-one with people whose physical constraints required a more individualized approach: patients recovering from joint replacements, people with severe balance deficits, adults in their eighties who had been sedentary for years and wanted to change that.

His teaching approach is grounded in a single conviction: that the body at any age responds to appropriate, consistent movement. Not to dramatic intervention. Not to punishment. To the kind of slow, deliberate, breath-coordinated practice that Tai Chi represents at its core. He has seen this conviction validated too many times to hold it lightly.

He holds decades of attention to how older bodies move, what helps them, and what does not. This book is an attempt to make that attention available to people who cannot be in the same room with him.

He lives simply and practices every morning, usually before the day has fully started.